Training Load in Professional Soccer

José M. Oliva Lozano • Luca P. Ardigò
Editors

Training Load in Professional Soccer

Guide to Monitoring Performance

Springer

Editors
José M. Oliva Lozano
United States Soccer Federation
Chicago, IL
USA

Luca P. Ardigò
Department of Teacher Education
NLA University College
Oslo, Norway

ISBN 978-3-031-52086-0 ISBN 978-3-031-52087-7 (eBook)
https://doi.org/10.1007/978-3-031-52087-7

This Springer imprint is published by the registered company Springer Nature Switzerland AG
The registered company address is: Gewerbestrasse 11, 6330 Cham, Switzerland

Preface

Soccer is the most popular sport in the world, and soccer research is a major field of interest among soccer scientists. Recently, a bibliometric review by Kirkendall and Krustrup (2022) of the existing literature revealed that from 1970 to 2019 nearly 17.000 scientific articles have been published based on a search in the Web of Science. Of these, 6000 examined professional soccer and from the millennium there has been an exponential increase in the number of publications. Thus, the immense international interest and commercial value of the game are reflected by high activity in the academic community.

Soccer is a hybrid sport combining endurance, repeated intense exercise, and explosive/ballistic actions with challenging cognition and coordination skills. Therefore, training in soccer is complex and requires a multifaceted approach. Most elite soccer teams therefore separate the sessions on the field into subcategories prioritizing perceptual, technical, and tactical elements, while also having a specific physiological aim. This requires thorough and qualified monitoring of the training load, as well as basic understanding of what training load is. For decades heart rate measurements have been the gold standard for measuring the cardiovascular loading in training in soccer, since heart rate is a good reflection of the oxygen uptake also during intermittent exercise. Also, different self-perceived methods such as rate of perceived exertion have been a standard tool to assess the load of training from a subjective angle. Thus, cardiovascular loading and subjective loading in training can be assessed with simple methods that are accessible to most teams.

However, today all teams at the elite and competitive level additionally apply tracking data based on GPS recordings, radio technology, multiple camera systems, and/or accelerometers as a reflection of the external training load. As there are many tracking systems, there are additionally, multiple suggestions of how to apply the data and to use it for a measure of physical loading. However, since tracking data are founded on external measures these should be interpreted with care. In the initial phase, tracking data were mostly focusing on total distance covered in training as a global measure of the training session, while distance covered in different high-speed running categories was used as indicators of anaerobic work. However, since the tracking technology advanced accelerations, decelerations and changes of directions performed within different thresholds are added as markers of speed, strength, and ballistic movements in training.

Since tracking data are external markers that are being translated into physiological loading, it is important and necessary to study the link between real physiological loading and the applied tracking indicators. This has to a certain degree been done during games by our research group, where statistical relationships have established between total game distance, as well as the ability to work during the last 15 min of a game, and skeletal muscle maximal activity in HAD, being a marker of β-oxidative capacity. Thus, total game distance and performance in the late stage of a game appear to reflect the ability of skeletal muscle to utilize fat as fuel. Moreover, we have seen similar inter-individual associations between the protein expression of skeletal muscle ion transporters in both male and female elite players and the ability to carry out high intensity running in games, while the number of type II fibers seems to reflect the ability to perform sprints and ballistic actions. These studies from games indicate that the tracking variables used to quantify game load have physiological value, but similar studies from training in elite soccer are currently warranted in the literature.

A highly debated area in soccer research as well in the practical community is the use of individual thresholds when quantifying the training load. Since a myriad of studies have provided evidence of large individual variations in game and training load, as well as differences in physical capacity, it has been suggested to adopt the thresholds of different tracking parameters to the individual player. This is a highly complicated task, and more research is needed in the area.

Going back to the bibliometric review recently by Kirkendall and Krustrup (2022), they also report the gender distribution in soccer research during the last 50 years. The authors demonstrate that for every paper published on women´s soccer there are six papers on the men´s game. Moreover, when looking solely at research in elite players with a focus on competitive indicators, such as training load, the distribution is even greater in favor of men. Thus, there is a large gender inequality in soccer research, and future studies on the application and development of training load protocols in elite soccer should prioritize women players to balance scientific information and reduce the risk of bias from purely adopting research done on males to women soccer athletes.

The evolution of soccer is moving fast, and the elite soccer in the future will be markedly more physically and mentally demanding than it is today. We recently analyzed the development in various variables such as time spend on games and training, intensity, and frequency of games during the last few decades, and we see a consistent increase, which is likely to evolve even further over the next decades. Also, the risk of injury is increasing in elite soccer. Thus, better qualified methods to record, measure, and interpret training and game load and to utilize technology in the daily management of players will become paramount in the future of elite and competitive soccer. Therefore, works such as the present one are highly important.

Magni Mohr
Centre of Health Sciences, Faculty of Health
University of the Faroe Islands
Tórshavn, Faroe Islands

Department of Sports Science and Clinical Biomechanics
SDU Sport and Health Sciences Cluster (SHSC)
Faculty of Health Sciences, University of Southern Denmark
Odense, Denmark

Acknowledgment

We would like to acknowledge and give our warmest thanks to all authors who made this book possible.

Contents

1 Definition and Context of Training Load

José M. Oliva Lozano, Ryan Curtis, and Vincenzo Rago

Training is considered the process of preparing athletes, physically, physiologically, psychologically, technically, and tactically, for the greatest possible level of performance (DeWeese et al. 2015; Stone et al. 2007). Training induces a psychophysiological response, which provides the stimulus for adaptation and depends on the nature, duration, and intensity of exercise (Viru and Viru 2000). Thus, coaches and applied sport scientists are increasingly taking scientific approaches to design and monitor training programs (Halson 2014). In this context, training load (TL) has been defined as the amount and intensity of exercise completed by the player (i.e., external load) and its associated internal response (i.e., internal load) (Wallace et al. 2014).

In general, TL monitoring allows practitioners to have a better understanding of the players' acute and chronic responses to the training program and competitive schedule. This information may provide a useful objective marker of physical performance output, which plays a key role in managing the overall training process (Impellizzeri et al. 2019; Oliva-Lozano et al. 2021). Specifically, TL monitoring has become important nowadays given that teams play a large number of matches during the season and congested schedules are experienced (i.e., teams may play three matches within 7–10 days) (Anderson et al. 2016; Palucci-Vieira et al. 2018).

J. M. Oliva Lozano (✉)
United States Soccer Federation, Chicago, IL, USA
e-mail: jol908@ual.es

R. Curtis
Korey Stringer Institute, University of Connecticut, Storrs, CT, USA

V. Rago
Physical Performance Department, Al Ain Football Club, Abu Dhabi, United Arab Emirates

J. M. Oliva Lozano, L. P. Ardigò (eds.), *Training Load in Professional Soccer*,
https://doi.org/10.1007/978-3-031-52087-7_1

1.1 External Load

External load describes the amount of exercise performed (Jaspers et al. 2017; Oliva-Lozano and Rago 2020) such as the duration of a session, distance covered at different speeds, accelerations, decelerations, sprints, or any specific measure of a player's movement (e.g., jumps, collisions, etc.). In this regard, player tracking technologies have led to a change in training load monitoring since these instruments provide a multitude of performance variables (Cummins et al. 2013; Pino-Ortega et al. 2021).

Data collected objectively from player tracking technologies can enhance training prescription through greater levels of individualization based on objective data. Each player has their own unique profile and characteristics (e.g., medical history, age, playing experience, and position), which should be used for context when interpreting the data.

1.2 Internal Load

Internal load represents the psychophysiological response (e.g., ratings of perceived exertion, oxygen consumption, heart rate, or lactate concentrations) induced by external training load (Gabbett 2016; Halson 2014; Impellizzeri et al. 2019). Regardless of the quantification method, strength and conditioning coaches usually prescribe training strategies according to external load in order to elicit a specific psychophysiological response (Impellizzeri et al. 2019). For instance, external training load is decreased as match day approaches (e.g., 2 days before or the day before the match) Oliva-Lozano et al. 2021, 2022, which reduces the stress of training before competition (Fessi et al. 2016).

Since internal load is ultimately the determinant of the training outcome and the driver of adaptation, it has been suggested that it should be used as a primary indicator for load monitoring (Impellizzeri et al. 2019). If similar external load is experienced by all the players from a squad, this does not imply that the internal load is going to be similar as well (Oliva-Lozano and Rago 2020). The internal load may vary according to contextual variables such as health status, fitness, genetics, or psychological factors (Impellizzeri et al. 2019; Vellers et al. 2018). Therefore, even having the same external load, players may experience different internal loads, and consequently, their adaptation to the stimulus may be different. In addition, several environmental variables (e.g. weather conditions) as well as match-related contextual variables (e.g., match outcome) (Rago et al. 2019) may affect the internal response to training (Impellizzeri et al. 2019).

Currently, the evolution of player tracking systems has increased the interest of sport scientist and coaches in external more so than internal load monitoring (Impellizzeri et al. 2019). Thus, practitioners are recommended to analyze the relationship between internal and external load since this relationship differs depending on the mode of training (McLaren et al. 2018).

1.3 The Player Monitoring Cycle

Given the relationship between load, injury, and performance, the player monitoring cycle has become increasingly important in the high-performance context (Gabbett et al. 2017). Gabbett et al. (2017) summarized this cycle based on four steps. First, external load needs to be quantified because coaches need to know what the player did. Second, coaches need to know what the internal response to that load was (i.e., internal load). Third, coaches should check if the player is tolerating the load (i.e., perceptual well-being). Fourth, it is important to analyze the physical and mental condition in order to know if the player is ready for the following stimuli (i.e., readiness to train or compete). By combining these steps, the player monitoring cycle may be understood as follows:

- Relationship between external and internal load. On the one hand, a player who experiences high external load may result in an increase in their internal load. Therefore, the coach may consider decreasing the load. However, if the internal load and external load were low, an increase in load may be necessary. On the other hand, if the external load was high and the internal load was low, this may mean that the player is already adapted to that training stimuli. Please note that maladaptive training responses may also be encountered (e.g., if the external load was low and internal load was high).
- Relationship between workload and perceptual well-being. In addition, the perceptual well-being may be useful to determine if the player is coping with the load. If the workload and perceptual well-being are high, the player may continue training/playing. If the workload is low but the perceptual well-being is high, it may be important to increase the workload. However, if the workload is high but the perceptual well-being is low, the coach may need to decrease the workload. Also, additional factors other than low or high workload may lead to poor well-being. Then, it would be necessary a qualitative analysis regarding the lifestyle, social or family issues, language difficulties, adaptation to the team, etc.
- Relationship between perceptual well-being and readiness. Finally, additional variables are analyzed to assess the level of readiness through submaximal stress tests or lower or upper body power tests, among others. If the perceptual well-being score is good and the readiness is high, the player may be ready to train/play. However, if the perceptual well-being and readiness are low, maybe, the player is not ready to train and requires additional recovery. Also, it is important to know that if the level of readiness is good but perceptual well-being is low, the player may need to increase mental preparation. Finally, if the perceptual well-being is high but readiness is poor, then the player may need to increase physical preparation.

However, this is not a perfect cycle. Although the importance of player load monitoring is understood, it is by no means an easy process to apply due to several contextual variables associated (Oliva-Lozano and Rago 2020). Player load monitoring in team sports have additional difficulties. For example, the principle of load individualization is difficult to apply because the player cannot be removed from the group/session so easily. Also, there are other tactical, technical, and coordinative variables, which may have influence. Thus, new research that adds physiological (e.g., changes in oxygen consumption), morphological, or technical-tactical (e.g., game model or playing positions) responses or adaptations to this process needs to be considered too.

References

Anderson L, Orme P, Di Michele R, Close GL, Morgans R, Drust B, Morton JP (2016) Quantification of training load during one-, two- and three-game week schedules in professional soccer players from the English premier league: implications for carbohydrate periodisation. J Sports Sci 34(13):1250–1259. https://doi.org/10.1080/02640414.2015.1106574

Cummins C, Orr R, O'Connor H, West C (2013) Global positioning systems and microtechnology sensors in team sports: a systematic review. Sports Med 43(10):1025–1042. https://doi.org/10.1007/s40279-013-0069-2

DeWeese BH, Hornsby G, Stone M, Stone MH (2015) The training process: planning for strength–power training in track and field. Part 1: theoretical aspects. J Sport Health Sci 4(4):308–317. https://doi.org/10.1016/j.jshs.2015.07.003

Fessi MS, Zarrouk N, Di Salvo V, Filetti C, Barker AR, Moalla W (2016) Effects of tapering on physical match activities in professional soccer players. J Sports Sci 34(24):2189–2194. https://doi.org/10.1080/02640414.2016.1171891

Gabbett TJ (2016) The training—injury prevention paradox: should athletes be training smarter and harder? Br J Sports Med 50(5):273–280. https://doi.org/10.1136/bjsports-2015-095788

Gabbett TJ, Nassis GP, Oetter E, Pretorius J, Johnston N, Medina D, Rodas G, Myslinski T, Howells D, Beard A, Ryan A (2017) The athlete monitoring cycle: a practical guide to interpreting and applying training monitoring data. Br J Sports Med 51(20):1451–1452. https://doi.org/10.1136/bjsports-2016-097298

Halson SL (2014) Monitoring training load to understand fatigue in athletes. Sports Med 44(2):139–147. https://doi.org/10.1007/s40279-014-0253-z

Impellizzeri FM, Marcora SM, Coutts AJ (2019) Internal and external training load: 15 years on. Int J Sports Physiol Perform 14(2):270–273. https://doi.org/10.1123/ijspp.2018-0935

Jaspers A, Brink MS, Probst SGM, Frencken WGP, Helsen WF (2017) Relationships between training load indicators and training outcomes in professional soccer. Sports Med 47(3):533–544. https://doi.org/10.1007/s40279-016-0591-0

McLaren SJ, Macpherson TW, Coutts AJ, Hurst C, Spears IR, Weston M (2018) The relationships between internal and external measures of training load and intensity in team sports: a meta-analysis. Sports Med 48(3):641–658. https://doi.org/10.1007/s40279-017-0830-z

Oliva-Lozano JM, Gómez-Carmona CD, Fortes V, Pino-Ortega J (2022) Effect of training day, match, and length of the microcycle on workload periodization in professional soccer players: a full-season study. Biol Sport 39(2):397–406

Oliva-Lozano JM, Gómez-Carmona CD, Rojas-Valverde D, Fortes V, Pino-Ortega J (2021) Effect of training day, match, and length of the microcycle on the worst-case scenarios in professional soccer players. Res Sports Med 1–14:425. https://doi.org/10.1080/15438627.2021.1895786

Oliva-Lozano JM, Muyor JM, Fortes V, McLaren SJ (2021) Decomposing the variability of match physical performance in professional soccer: implications for monitoring individuals. Eur J Sport Sci 21(11):1588–1596. https://doi.org/10.1080/17461391.2020.1842513

Oliva-Lozano JM, Rago V (2020) El Sport Scientist y la monitorización de la carga con EPTS en deportes de equipo. Editorial Universidad de Almería, Almería

Palucci-Vieira LH, Aquino R, Lago-Peñas C, Munhoz-Martins GH, Puggina EF, Barbieri FA, Palucci Vieira LH, Aquino R, Lago-Peñas C, Munhoz Martins GH, Puggina EF, Barbieri

FA (2018) Running performance in Brazilian professional football players during a congested match schedule. J Strength Cond Res 32(2):313–325. https://doi.org/10.1519/JSC.0000000000002342

Pino-Ortega J, Oliva-Lozano JM, Gantois P, Nakamura FY, Rico-González M (2021) Comparison of the validity and reliability of local positioning systems against other tracking technologies in team sport: a systematic review. Proc Inst Mech Eng P: J Sports Eng Technol 175433712098823:73. https://doi.org/10.1177/1754337120988236

Rago V, Rebelo A, Krustrup P, Mohr M (2019) Contextual variables and training load throughout a competitive period in a top-level male soccer team. J Strength Cond Res 1–7:3177. https://doi.org/10.1519/jsc.0000000000003258

Stone M, Sands W, Stone M (2007) Principles and practice of strength-power training. Human Kinetics, Champaign, IL

Vellers HL, Kleeberger SR, Lightfoot JT (2018) Inter-individual variation in adaptations to endurance and resistance exercise training: genetic approaches towards understanding a complex phenotype. Mamm Genome 29(1–2):48–62. https://doi.org/10.1007/s00335-017-9732-5

Viru A, Viru M (2000) Nature of training effects. In: Garrett WE, Kirkendall DT (eds) Exercise and sport science. Lippincott Williams & Wilkins, Philadelphia, PA, pp 67–95

Wallace LK, Slattery KM, Coutts AJ (2014) A comparison of methods for quantifying training load: relationships between modelled and actual training responses. Eur J Appl Physiol 114(1):11–20. https://doi.org/10.1007/s00421-013-2745-1

Methods for Monitoring Training Load

2

José M. Oliva Lozano, José M. Muyor, José Pino-Ortega, and Luca P. Ardigò

As mentioned in the first chapter, training load monitoring helps to make evidence-based decisions to decrease the injury risk and optimize player's performance. Many soccer teams (especially at the top level) employ sport scientists who engage in this role on a daily basis (Akenhead and Nassis 2016). However, current developments in technology have allowed sport scientists to monitor training load using various methods.

2.1 Methods for Monitoring Internal Load

2.1.1 Rating of Perceived Exertion (RPE)

Although new apps are now available to measure RPE, this may be considered as the simplest method to quantify the internal load since it is a practical, noninvasive, and cheap method (Impellizzeri et al. 2004; Wallace et al. 2014). For instance, the

J. M. Oliva Lozano (✉)
United States Soccer Federation, Chicago, IL, USA
e-mail: jol908@ual.es

J. M. Muyor
Health Research Centre, University of Almería, Almería, Spain

Laboratory of Kinesiology, Biomechanics and Ergonomics (KIBIOMER Lab), Research Central Services, University of Almería, Almería, Spain

J. Pino-Ortega
Physical Activity and Sports Department, Faculty of Sports Science, University of Murcia, San Javier, Murcia, Spain

L. P. Ardigò
Department of Teacher Education, NLA University College, Oslo, Norway
e-mail: luca.ardigo@nla.no

J. M. Oliva Lozano, L. P. Ardigò (eds.), *Training Load in Professional Soccer*, https://doi.org/10.1007/978-3-031-52087-7_2

"Borg scale" (Borg 1998) associates the perceived exertion of the player in a session with values between 6 and 20, considering 6 as no exertion at all and 20 as maximal exertion (Table 2.1).

However, it may be complex for the player to accurately rate the perceived exertion with a 15-grade scale, and therefore, other simpler scales such as the CR-10, which is also known as the "modified Borg scale," were developed (Arney et al. 2019; Wilson and Jones 1989). This is a 10-grade scale (Table 2.2) which has significant practical implications for coaches since previous research showed that after 6, the second ventilatory threshold (i.e., anaerobic threshold) was found in professional soccer players (Algrøy et al. 2011). Furthermore, another advantage is that it is a psychophysiological scale (Abbiss et al. 2015), which can be applied retrospectively and measure RPE even 48 h after the session (Fanchini et al. 2017). In addition, RPE may be multiplied by the total duration of the session, which is known as the session-RPE and serves as another method to quantify training load (Foster et al. 2001).

Table 2.1 Borg scale (Borg 1998)

Ratings	Description
6	No exertion at all
7	Extremely light
8	
9	Very light
10	
11	Light
12	
13	Somewhat hard
14	
15	Hard
16	
17	Very hard
18	
19	Extremely hard
20	Maximal exertion

Table 2.2 Modified Borg scale (Wilson and Jones 1989)

Ratings	Description
0	Nothing at all
1	Very very slight
2	Very slight
3	Moderate
4	Somewhat severe
5	Severe
6	
7	Very severe
8	
9	Very very severe
10	Maximal

However, one of the main limitations of RPE as a method to quantify internal load is that it is a subjective method (Chen et al. 2002). Coaches need to consider that there is a risk of false ratings reported by the players, especially with professional players, who depend on their performance to keep their professional role (Oliva-Lozano and Rago 2020). For example, if one player is fatigued or cannot perform at his/her best level and his/her RPE is very high, the player might lie (Oliva-Lozano and Rago 2020). This does not mean that the player wants to deceive us, but he/she knows that this information might generate the suspicion of poor shape or that there is another player in better fit to replace him/her in the competition (Oliva-Lozano and Rago 2020). Also, there is a lack of consensus on (a) when and how to ask the question to the athlete regarding the perceived exertion effort and (b) which word should be assigned to each category of exertion (Oliva-Lozano and Rago 2020). In addition, the RPE is based on a discontinuous scale which, technically, does not quantify the perceived exertion, but rather classifies it. This is why other methods such as the visual analog scale or the centiMax scale, which is also known as CR100, have been proposed (Borg and Borg 2002; Foster et al. 2021; Rebelo et al. 2012).

2.1.2 Heart Rate Monitoring

The development of heart rate monitors has allowed to monitor heart rate during any physical activity. Heart rate monitoring is a useful method, especially when measuring the percentage of maximum heart rate, given that it is correlated with maximum oxygen consumption (VO_{2MAX}) (Achten and Jeukendrup 2003). It has become one of most common methods for internal load monitoring, and currently, coaches may get information about mean and maximum heart rate, heart rate reserve, percentage of time spent in each training zone (e.g., above 95% of maximum heart rate or heart rate reserve), heart rate variability, heart rate recovery, etc. Also, previous authors have suggested monitoring heart rate to RPE ratio, which may aid in explaining fatigue based on establishing a relationship between objective and subjective measures (Halson 2014; Martin and Andersen 2000).

However, the main limitation of measuring heart rate is that the players need to wear heart rate monitors (usually with a chest band) and they may consider them somewhat invasive. Thus, the industry of performance tracking systems is trying to develop specific vests or t-shirts, which include the technology for heart rate monitoring (Pino-Ortega et al. 2019).

2.1.3 Biochemical/Hormonal/Immunological Assessments

In recent years, an increasing number of studies have been conducted regarding the biological response to exercise with special focus on the analysis of fatigue and performance optimization (Halson 2014; Nowakowska et al. 2019; Walker et al. 2019). Some biomarkers are blood lactate concentration, serum creatine kinase activity, salivary cortisol, testosterone, or salivary immunoglobin A. However, these methods of internal load monitoring are costly and time consuming yet to be applied in soccer (Halson 2014).

2.1.4 Sleep Monitoring

Poor sleep quality may have negative effects on performance, perception of effort, motivation, and various biological functions (Halson 2014; Nédélec et al. 2015). Given that sleep provides physiological and psychological functions which are key for optimal recovery, suboptimal sleeping patterns may lead to impaired recovery in professional soccer players (Nédélec et al. 2015). Therefore, it is important to monitor sleep quality and quantity for early detection and treatment before significant performance decrements are observed (Halson 2014). Coaches may use simple diaries or questionnaires that indicate the total hours of sleep and perceived sleep quality. Nonetheless, new methods based on inertial sensors (e.g., accelerometers) may be of interest for coaches since more detailed information is provided (e.g., bedtime, wake time or sleep efficiency, etc.)

2.1.5 Other Questionnaires and Diaries

These are simple methods to keep collecting internal load variables such as wellness, mood states, or recovery. For this reason, there is a number of questionnaires available, which include the Daily Analysis of Life Demands for Athletes (DALDA) (Rushall 1990), the Total Quality of Recovery (TQR) scale (Kenttä and Hassmén 1998), or Profile of Mood States (POMS) (Lovell et al. 2010; McNair et al. 1971), among others. However, coaches need to avoid "questionnaire fatigue" by considering a proper length of the questionnaire and frequency of questionnaire administration (Halson 2014).

2.2 Methods for Monitoring External Load

Traditionally, external load monitoring was based on training volume considering the total duration of the session (e.g., training/playing minutes) or the total number of sessions/matches experienced by the player within the microcycle. However, developments in technology have allowed to access new methods for external load monitoring. For example, currently, electronic performance and tracking systems (EPTS) are becoming the most common methods for time-motion analysis in soccer, especially at elite levels. EPTS track the player positioning on the field and a plethora of variables (e.g., distance covered, total of accelerations and decelerations, total of high-speed actions, maximum speed, etc.) are collected. Specifically, some EPTS usually include inertial measurement units (e.g., accelerometers, gyroscopes, or magnetometers) that allow the collection of triaxial load parameters such as jumps, horizontal body impacts, landings, or specific measures of goalkeeper's load (e.g., right dives, left dives, G-force absorbed by the goalkeeper when diving, stance time, etc.). In addition, these may be used in combination with physiological sensors (e.g., heart rate monitors), which collect internal load variables.

Although combinations between EPTS may exist, there are three main forms of EPTS available in the market (Oliva-Lozano and Rago 2020):

(a) Global navigation satellite systems (GNSS): these EPTS require that the players wear a tracking unit, which connects to the satellite constellations, and positioning may be calculated (Fig. 2.1). These EPTS highly depend on a successful connection between the receiver (i.e., tracking unit) and the satellites, which implies that it is not possible to collect data or get a good signal (e.g., indoor facilities). However, these EPTS are easy to use, usually cheaper than other forms of EPTS, and are composed of physiological and inertial sensors.

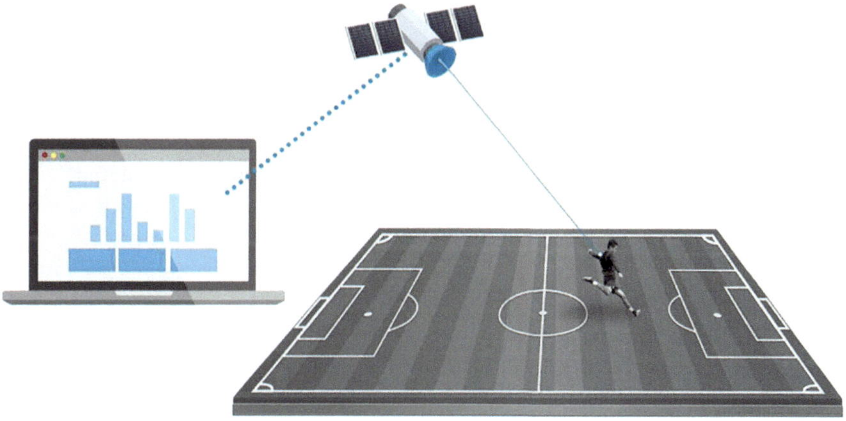

Fig. 2.1 Use of global navigation satellite systems in soccer

(b) Local positioning systems (LPS): these EPTS were applied to soccer mainly as a consequence of the limitations to collect data in some stadiums through GNSS in addition to the validity and reliability limitations of this technology. LPS use multiple antennas, which are placed in the stadium surrounding the pitch, to collect player positioning (Fig. 2.2). The use of LPS is similar to GNSS-based EPTS since both require the player to wear a tracking unit, collect similar variables, and may be combined with physiological and inertial sensors. In addition, some EPTS combine both GNSS and LPS technologies, which allow player load monitoring in outdoor locations using GNSS and indoor venues (e.g., domes or stadiums with limited coverage for GNSS). However, previous installation is required and the financial investment is relatively high.

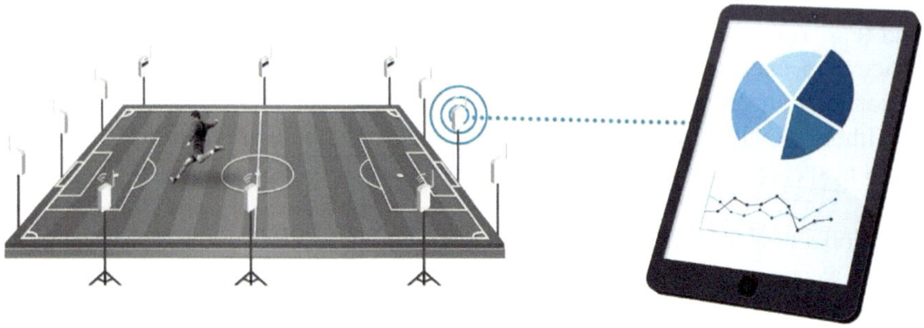

Fig. 2.2 Use of local positioning systems in soccer

(c) Optical tracking systems (OTS): these EPTS are based on specific tracking cameras which are set in the stadiums to record the positioning of the players and the ball (Fig. 2.3). The main advantage of these EPTS is that the players do not need to wear any tracking device. However, the cost and complexity of installation are usually greater compared to other EPTS (Curtis et al. 2019; Oliva-Lozano and Rago 2020). In this regard, it is important to mention that the use of these EPTS is usually specific to match day. In addition, external load variables such as body impacts or jumps, which are collected by inertial sensors, or internal load variables (e.g., mean heart rate) are not registered.

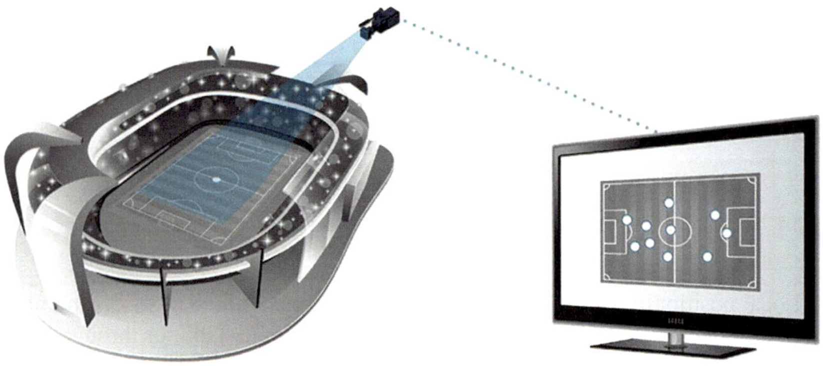

Fig. 2.3 Use of optical tracking systems in soccer

Moreover, data collected by these EPTS may be also used for real-time analysis. Therefore, the staff may have access to player load during a specific training session or match and make decisions based on this information. For instance, coaches may compare real-time data to the training objectives and adjust the session intensity and/or volume accordingly (Weaving et al. 2017).

Also, although all these EPTS provide coaches with external load monitoring data, these may be used for tactical purposes (e.g., measuring team width or team length). Nonetheless, the validity and reliability of GNSS technology may be questionable for this purpose. For instance, a recent study showed that the mean spatial measurement error of GNSS was ~96 cm, which was greater than OTS (~56 cm) and LPS (~23 cm) (Linke et al. 2018).

References

Abbiss CR, Peiffer JJ, Meeusen R, Skorski S (2015) Role of ratings of perceived exertion during self-paced exercise: what are we actually measuring? Sports Med 45(9):1235–1243. https://doi.org/10.1007/s40279-015-0344-5

Achten J, Jeukendrup AE (2003) Heart rate monitoring. Sports Med 33(7):517–538. https://doi.org/10.2165/00007256-200333070-00004

Akenhead R, Nassis GP (2016) Training load and player monitoring in high-level football: current practice and perceptions. Int J Sports Physiol Perform 11(5):587–593. https://doi.org/10.1123/ijspp.2015-0331

Algrøy EA, Hetlelid KJ, Seiler S, Pedersen JIS (2011) Quantifying training intensity distribution in a group of Norwegian professional soccer players. Int J Sports Physiol Perform 6(1):70–81. https://doi.org/10.1123/ijspp.6.1.70

Arney BE, Glover R, Fusco A, Cortis C, de Koning JJ, van Erp T, Jaime S, Mikat RP, Porcari JP, Foster C (2019) Comparison of RPE (rating of perceived exertion) scales for session RPE. Int J Sports Physiol Perform 14(7):994–996. https://doi.org/10.1123/ijspp.2018-0637

Borg G (1998) Borg's perceived exertion and pain scales. Human Kinetics, Champaign, IL

Borg E, Borg G (2002) A comparison of AME and CR100 for scaling perceived exertion. Acta Psychol 109(2):157–175. https://doi.org/10.1016/S0001-6918(01)00055-5

Chen MJ, Fan X, Moe ST (2002) Criterion-related validity of the Borg ratings of perceived exertion scale in healthy individuals: a meta-analysis. J Sports Sci 20(11):873–899. https://doi.org/10.1080/026404102320761787

Curtis R, Courteney B, Huggins R, Casa DJ (2019) Elite soccer players: maximizing performance and safety. Routledge, London

Fanchini M, Ferraresi I, Petruolo A, Azzalin A, Ghielmetti R, Schena F, Impellizzeri FM (2017) Is a retrospective RPE appropriate in soccer? Response shift and recall bias. Sci Med Footb 1(1):53–59. https://doi.org/10.1080/02640414.2016.1231411

Foster C, Boullosa D, McGuigan M, Fusco A, Cortis C, Arney BE, Orton B, Dodge C, Jaime S, Radtke K, van Erp T, de Koning JJ, Bok D, Rodriguez-Marroyo JA, Porcari JP (2021) 25 years of session rating of perceived exertion: historical perspective and development. Int J Sports Physiol Perform 16(5):612–621. https://doi.org/10.1123/ijspp.2020-0599

Foster C, Florhaug JA, Franklin J, Gottschall L, Hrovatin LA, Parker S, Doleshal P, Dodge C (2001) A new approach to monitoring exercise training. J Strength Cond Res 15(1):109–115. https://doi.org/10.1519/00124278-200102000-00019

Halson SL (2014) Monitoring training load to understand fatigue in athletes. Sports Med 44(2):139–147. https://doi.org/10.1007/s40279-014-0253-z

Impellizzeri F, Rampinini E, Coutts AJ, Sassi A, Marcora SM (2004) Use of RPE-based training load in soccer. Med Sci Sports Exerc 36(6):1042–1047. https://doi.org/10.1249/01.MSS.0000128199.23901.2F

Kenttä G, Hassmén P (1998) Overtraining and recovery. Sports Med 26(1):1–16. https://doi.org/10.2165/00007256-199826010-00001

Linke D, Link D, Lames M (2018) Validation of electronic performance and tracking systems EPTS under field conditions. PLoS One 13(7):1–19. https://doi.org/10.1371/journal.pone.0199519

Lovell G, Townrow J, Thatcher R (2010) Mood states of soccer players in the English leagues: reflections of an increasing workload. Biol Sport 27(2):83–88. https://doi.org/10.5604/20831862.913072

Martin DT, Andersen MB (2000) Heart rate-perceived exertion relationship during training and taper. J Sports Med Phys Fitness 40(3):201–208. http://www.ncbi.nlm.nih.gov/pubmed/11125762

McNair DM, Lorr M, Droppelman LE (1971) Manual for the profile of mood states. Educational and Industrial Testing Services, Princeton, NJ

Nédélec M, Halson S, Abaidia A-E, Ahmaidi S, Dupont G (2015) Stress, sleep and recovery in elite soccer: a critical review of the literature. Sports Med 45(10):1387–1400. https://doi.org/10.1007/s40279-015-0358-z

Nowakowska A, Kostrzewa-Nowak D, Buryta R, Nowak R (2019) Blood biomarkers of recovery efficiency in soccer players. Int J Environ Res Public Health 16(18):1–28. https://doi.org/10.3390/ijerph16183279

Oliva-Lozano JM, Rago V (2020) El Sport Scientist y la monitorización de la carga con EPTS en deportes de equipo. Editorial Universidad de, Almería

Pino-Ortega J, Bastida-Castillo A, Oliva-Lozano JM, Rojas-Valverde D, Reche-Soto P, Gómez-Carmona C (2019) Comparison of two methods for recording heart rate telemetry: chest band vs technical shirt. Retos 36:469–473. https://recyt.fecyt.es/index.php/retos/article/view/68676

Rebelo A, Brito J, Seabra A, Oliveira J, Drust B, Krustrup P (2012) A new tool to measure training load in soccer training and match play. Int J Sports Med 33(4):297–304. https://doi.org/10.1055/s-0031-1297952

Rushall BS (1990) A tool for measuring stress tolerance in elite athletes. J Appl Sport Psychol 2(1):51–66. https://doi.org/10.1080/10413209008406420

Walker AJ, McFadden BA, Sanders DJ, Rabideau MM, Hofacker ML, Arent SM (2019) Biomarker response to a competitive season in division I female soccer players. J Strength Cond Res 33(10):2622–2628. https://doi.org/10.1519/JSC.0000000000003264

Wallace LK, Slattery KM, Impellizzeri FM, Coutts AJ (2014) Establishing the criterion validity and reliability of common methods for quantifying training load. J Strength Cond Res 28(8):2330–2337. https://doi.org/10.1519/JSC.0000000000000416

Weaving D, Whitehead S, Till K, Jones B (2017) Validity of real-time data generated by a wearable microtechnology device. J Strength Cond Res 31(10):2876–2879. https://doi.org/10.1519/JSC.0000000000002127

Wilson RC, Jones PW (1989) A comparison of the visual analogue scale and modified Borg scale for the measurement of dyspnoea during exercise. Clin Sci 76(3):277–282. https://doi.org/10.1042/cs0760277

3 Training Load Parameters in Soccer

Marcin Andrzejewski, Marek Konefał, Marco Beato, and Paweł Chmura

Training load monitoring in team sports is a challenging task because the physiological and mechanical demands vary depending on the type of activity, volume, intensity, and other contextual variables (Bangsbo et al. 2006; Marynowicz et al. 2020). Monitoring soccer players' training load is essential for determining whether they are adapting to their training program, understanding individual responses to training, assessing fatigue and the associated need for recovery, and minimizing the risk of nonfunctional overreaching, injury, and illness (Bourdon et al. 2017; Foster 1998; Gabbett 2016; Gabbett et al. 2014; Halson 2014; Owen et al. 2016). Research shows that accurate management of training load is also crucial for the planning and periodization of training (Little and Williams 2007). As mentioned in previous chapters, measures of training load can be categorized as either internal or external (Impellizzeri et al. 2019). The application of an external load induces a physiological response (i.e., internal load) providing input to the athlete's training stress-adaptation system.

M. Andrzejewski
Department of Methodology of Recreation, Poznań University of Physical Education, Poznań, Poland

M. Konefał
Department of Biological and Motor Sport Bases, Wroclaw University of Health and Sport Sciences, Wrocław, Poland

M. Beato
School of Health and Sports Sciences, University of Suffolk, Ipswich, UK

P. Chmura (✉)
Department of Team Games, Wroclaw University of Health and Sport Sciences, Wrocław, Poland

J. M. Oliva Lozano, L. P. Ardigò (eds.), *Training Load in Professional Soccer*, https://doi.org/10.1007/978-3-031-52087-7_3

For the context of this chapter internal training loads are defined as the relative biological (both physiological and psychological) stressors imposed on the athlete during training or competition (Bourdon et al. 2017). Measures such as heart rate (HR), blood lactate (La), oxygen consumption (VO_2), and ratings of perceived exertion (RPE) are commonly used to assess internal load (Scott et al. 2013). HR methods have been examined in individual sports and team sports. For example, the training impulse (TRIMP) is a HR-based method, converting the HR data from a training session into an arbitrary unit (AU) that reflects the physical effort (Jaspers et al. 2017). Another method used to study internal workload consists of multiplying the session rating of perceived exertion (RPE) by session duration (Foster et al. 2001), which is well known as training load (training $load_{RPE}$). In addition, some variations are examined such as weekly training $load_{RPE}$, weekly monotony (i.e., the daily mean of weekly training $load_{RPE}$ divided by the standard deviation), and weekly strain (i.e., the total weekly training $load_{RPE}$ multiplied by monotony) (Foster 1998). These parameters will be discussed in more detail later in this chapter.

On the other hand, common measures of external load can be collected by multiple tools such as electronic performance and tracking systems (e.g., global positioning systems, GPS; or video-based tracking technologies), foot sensors, encoders, and power meters (Aughey 2011; Beato et al. 2018; Cummins et al. 2013; Dellaserra et al. 2014). For example, the use of GPS is becoming increasingly common because of its great practicality (Burgess 2017; Johnston et al. 2013; Varley et al. 2012). Some of the metrics provided by this technology that practitioners can use to analyze activity profiles of athletes include total distance covered, distance covered at different speed zones, the number of accelerations and decelerations, metabolic power, and player load (Akenhead and Nassis 2016). In addition, different types of sensors are used for assessment of athletes' training intensity and internal load based on physiological and perceptual responses (e.g., rating of perceived exertion, heart rate, body temperature, sweat measures, salivary cortisol, muscle oxygen saturation, or muscle activation).

An integrated approach to training load is also important, and for this reason internal and external training loads should be used in combination to provide greater insight to training stress (Gabbett 2016). For example, soccer players repeating the exact same session on different days may maintain the same external load output for the same duration but experience quite different internal loads (heart rate, blood lactate, RPE, etc.) depending on their state of fatigue, emotional disturbances, recent training history, or illness. This uncoupling of internal and external loads may aid in determining the players' readiness (Bourdon et al. 2017; Halson 2014).

From a physiological perspective, if the external load is increased, it should lead to a greater internal load and metabolic stress (di Prampero et al. 1986; Wallace et al. 2014). This metabolic stress is related to muscle contractions, which mainly require the provision of oxygen in the case of aerobic energy-burning processes. These are primarily challenges to the cardiorespiratory system, and therefore, measures of internal physiological load are most often related to oxygen consumption and cardiac output.

3.1 Internal Training Load Parameters

3.1.1 Perception of Effort

The rating of perceived exertion (RPE) is one of the most common means of assessing internal load. The use of RPE is based on the notion that an athlete can monitor their physiological stress during exercise as well as retrospectively provide information regarding their perceived effort post training or competition. Evidence suggests that RPE correlates well with heart rate during steady-state exercise and high-intensity interval cycling training, but not as well during short-duration high-intensity soccer drills (Borresen and Ian Lambert 2009). Further, a meta-analysis of the literature reported that while RPE is a valid means of assessing exercise intensity, the validity may not be as high as previously thought (Chen et al. 2002). For example, weighted mean validity coefficients for heart rate (HR), blood lactate, and percent of maximal oxygen uptake (VO_2max) were 0.62, 0.57, and 0.64, respectively (Chen et al. 2002). RPE is also often combined with other variables such as session duration, HR, and blood lactate to provide additional insights into the internal load experienced by the athlete (Halson 2014).

3.1.2 Session Rating of Perceived Exertion (RPE)

Foster (1998) developed the session-RPE method of quantifying training load, which involves multiplying the athlete's RPE (on a 1–10 scale) by the duration of the session (in minutes).

$$\text{Training load}\left(\text{a.u.}\right) = \text{RPE} \times \text{session duration}\left(\text{min}\right)$$

where training load is training load, a.u. is arbitrary units, and RPE is the rating of perceived exertion.

This simple method has been shown to be valid and reliable, with individual correlations between session-RPE and summated HR zone scores ranging between $r = 0.75$ and $r = 0.90$ (Foster 1998). Subsequent research in soccer training has identified individual correlations between RPE and HR zones (ranging from $r = 0.54$ to $r = 0.78$) and a correlation of $r = 0.84$ has also been reported in endurance athletes (Borresen and Lambert 2008).

The "monotony" and "strain" indexes can also be calculated from session-RPE method data of a training microcycle (Clemente 2019). The training monotony is a measure of day-to-day training variability that has been found to be related to the onset of overtraining when monotonous training is combined with high training loads (Foster 1998). Training monotony is calculated using the following formula:

$$\text{Monotony} = \text{weekly mean training load} \div \text{standard deviation of weekly training load}$$

Another score that might be a useful unit for monitoring training when players are undertaking high training loads is the training strain. This variable is equal to the multiplication of the weekly training load and the monotony scores. Recovery only becomes fundamental to training when high training loads are being undertaken; therefore, the calculation of training strain appears advantageous. For example, when training loads are high and there has been low variability of load (resulting in a high monotony index), the training strain is high. This type of training has been associated with the incidence of illness and poor performance (Putlur et al. 2004). Conversely, training strain is low when players complete either high or low training loads with regular variation in load sessions (i.e., low monotony). In general, high levels of training strain are usually only reached during the preparation period of training when there is no regular competition.

$$\text{Training strain} = \text{weekly training load} \times \text{monotony}$$

The session-RPE method was developed to eliminate the need to utilize HR monitors or other methods of assessing exercise intensity. While the session-RPE method may be simple, valid, and reliable, the addition of HR monitoring may aid in understanding some of the variance that it does not explain.

3.1.3 Heart Rate (HR) to RPE Ratio

HR is one of the most common markers of internal load. The use of HR monitoring during exercise is based on the linear relationship between HR and the rate of oxygen consumption during steady-state exercise (Haddad et al. 2017; Hopkins 1991), where the percentage of maximum HR is often used to both prescribe and monitor intensity (Borresen and Lambert 2008). HR can be used with many forms to monitor training load and one of them is the percentage of maximal HR (%HRmax) observed during exercise. Examination of physiological and perceptual indicators of load at a fixed submaximal intensity can provide information on the state of fatigue of the athlete. The combination of HR and perception of effort measures (HR–RPE ratio) may aid in elucidating fatigue (Martin and Andersen 2000). For example, the internal load of a cyclist who has a reduced submaximal HR in combination with an elevated RPE may be quite different from a cyclist with a normal HR–RPE ratio (Pyne and Martin 2011). Moreover, strong and very strong correlations were found between the session-RPE method and %HRmax during soccer-specific training sessions and during Australian football sessions, for instance (Scott et al. 2013).

3.1.4 Training Impulse (TRIMP)

Bannister's training impulse (TRIMP) is a method used to quantify training load. It is calculated with a pre-evaluated coefficient obtained with the relationship between HR and blood lactate during an incremental exercise (y), multiplied with the HR reserve (HRres) and the duration of the sessions (t) (Banister 1991). Its use was correlated to the session-RPE method during soccer training and match (Alexiou and Coutts 2008; Foster et al. 2001).

Edwards' TRIMP is a method used for the calculation of training load with the time spent in five arbitrary HR zones multiplied by arbitrary coefficient (>50–60% ×1, >60–70% ×2, >70–80% ×3, >80–90% ×4, >90–100% ×5) (Edwards 1993). This method was not validated with a known physiological response but was used in several studies as a good indicator of training load.

Lucia's TRIMP is also a method used to measure training load related to the ventilatory thresholds (VT1 and VT2). VT1 corresponds to the anaerobic threshold and VT2 to the respiratory compensation threshold. This method provides three zones, low (<VT1), moderate (VT1–VT2), and high (>VT2), and each zone corresponds to a coefficient: 1, 2, and 3 respectively. Training load is calculated with the time spent in each zone multiplied by the corresponding coefficient and added to each other (Lucia et al. 2003). Its use was correlated to the session-RPE method during soccer and swimming training sessions (Alexiou and Coutts 2008; Wallace et al. 2009).

The oxygen uptake during exercise (VO_2) and its expression as percentage of the maximal volume of oxygen uptake ($\%VO_{2max}$) were both strongly correlated to the session-RPE method for males and females practicing interval training (Wallace et al. 2014).

3.1.5 Lactate (La)

Blood lactate concentration (La) is sensitive to changes in exercise intensity and duration (Beneke et al. 2011); however, there are a number of potential limitations to the use of regular monitoring of lactate concentrations during training and competition. These include inter- and intraindividual differences in lactate accumulation depending on ambient temperature, hydration status, diet, glycogen content, previous exercise, and amount of muscle mass utilized, as well as sampling procedures (time and site) (Borresen and Lambert 2008).

Lactate threshold (LT) determination is one of the most relevant indicators of aerobic performance and training status. LT is where the pace has been raised to a point where Krebs cycle (aerobic energy), in muscle cells, cannot provide sufficient energy anymore. This threshold is usually observed at around 2 $mmol{\cdot}l^{-1}$. The second threshold, where a second increase in lactate accumulation happens around 4 $mmol{\cdot}l^{-1}$, is referred to as the onset of blood lactate threshold (OBLA). The velocities at LT (vLT) and OBLA (vOBLA) are the pace when running just before exceeding the LT and the OBLA point, respectively (Haddad et al. 2017). Their use was strongly correlated to the session-RPE method during soccer training sessions, for instance (Akubat et al. 2012). This shows that, like the HR–RPE ratio, the lactate to RPE ratio may be useful in determining internal load and identifying fatigue in athletes (Akubat et al. 2012). Again, changes in these parameters at a fixed submaximal workload may be useful to identify physiological and perceptual changes in internal load.

3.1.6 HR Recovery (HRR)

HR recovery (HRR) is the rate at which HR declines at the cessation of exercise and has been suggested to be a marker of autonomic function and training status in athletes (Daanen et al. 2012). The autonomic nervous system consists of the sympathetic and parasympathetic systems, with the rise in HR during exercise being the result of increased sympathetic activity in combination with a reduction in parasympathetic activity. HRR is characterized by opposing autonomic nervous system activity, with an increase in parasympathetic activity and withdrawal of sympathetic nervous activity (Shetler et al. 2001). HRR can be calculated over varying timeframes, usually between 30 s and 2 min, with the difference between end of exercise HR and HR at 60 s post-exercise being most commonly used (Daanen et al. 2012). In a recent review on HRR and monitoring changes in training status, it is suggested that HRR improves with increased training status, remains unchanged when there is no change in training status, and decreases when training status is reduced. It was then concluded that, with the exception of overreaching (where research is conflicting), HRR could be used to monitor the accumulation of fatigue in athletes (Daanen et al. 2012).

3.1.7 HR Variability (HRV)

The measurement of resting or post-exercise HR variability (HRV) has been suggested to indicate both positive and negative adaptations to training (Plews et al. 2013). However, the varying methodological approaches employed, as well as high day-to-day variability in environmental and homeostatic factors, have resulted in inconsistent findings in the scientific literature (Plews et al. 2013). As such, HRV has been shown to increase without a change in fitness (VO_2max) (Portier et al. 2001) as well as decrease alongside increases in fitness (Iellamo et al. 2002). Increases, decreases, and no change in HRV have also been reported in the overtraining literature (Halson and Jeukendrup 2004). To overcome some of the inconsistencies in findings, it has been suggested that both weekly and 7-day rolling averages have higher validity than single-day measurements (Plews et al. 2012). While various HRV indices can be measured, Plews et al. (2013) prefer the use of the natural logarithm of the square root of the mean sum of the squared differences between R–R intervals (Ln rMSSD). This is due to the lower coefficient of variation compared with other indices, a lack of influence of breathing frequency, and that data can be collected over a short period of time and easily calculated. As is the case with the majority of tools to monitor elite athletes, longitudinal monitoring and an understanding of individual responses in HRV to training, taper and competition are critical.

3.2 External Training Load Parameters

External load (EL) refers to any external stimulus applied to the player and will result in psychological and physiological responses (Halson 2014; Wallace et al. 2009). Measuring EL includes quantifying the training and competition load of a player, such as duration of a training session, the total distance covered (TDC), and number of high-intensity sprints (HIS) (Halson 2014; Soligard et al. 2016; Wallace et al. 2009). To gain an understanding of external training load, a number of technologies are available to athletes and coaches. In running-based team sports, one of the most valid and reliable tools for monitoring metrics related to external training load is the global positioning system (GPS) (Varley et al. 2012). The reliability of GPS for monitoring movement is influenced by factors such as sample rate, velocity, and duration and type of task (Aughey 2011; Beato and de Keijzer 2019). From the available literature, it appears that the higher the velocity of movement, the lower the GPS reliability (Aughey 2011). Further, the reliability is also reduced when assessing tasks that require a change of direction and GPS does not quantify the load of jumping, kicking the ball, and tackling actions (Aughey 2011). Use of this system is also becoming increasingly common because of its great practicality (Beato et al. 2018; Burgess 2017). Some of the metrics provided by this system that practitioners can use to analyze activity profiles of athletes include total distance covered, distance covered at different speed zones, the number of accelerations and decelerations, player load, and metabolic power (Akenhead and Nassis 2016; Reynolds et al. 2021).

3.2.1 Total Distance Covered and Distance per Minute

One of the first and most common parameters that we analyze in terms of external loads of soccer players is the total distance covered, which evaluates the "volume" of work performed by the player. This parameter allows the coaches to assess the total volume of work that the soccer players has performed during the match or training (Andrzejewski et al. 2016, 2018, 2019; Chmura et al. 2019). This parameter, of course, is only a baseline value, which requires a deeper analysis of the distance covered in the various intensity ranges (this will be discussed in the next paragraph). Since the total distance covered by a soccer player varies greatly depending on many context variables (such as position on the pitch, match outcome, location of the match being played, the quality of the opponent, weather conditions) (Andrzejewski et al. 2016; Chmura et al. 2018, 2021; Konefał et al. 2020, 2021) and many other reasons; therefore, we suggest that much more attention should be spent in the analysis of this parameter on the relative distance covered by the player ($m.min^{-1}$). Relative distance is simply the average distance an athlete travels per minute during training or competition. While total distance provides a clear picture of the athlete's volume, relative distance displays the "intensity." This value will allow a more detailed insight into the intensity that was developed by the player during a match, training, or specific exercise. It is important for sports scientists to understand the importance of monitoring and analyzing the relative distance traveled by a player, as this variation in the work pace pattern can significantly affect the level of players' fatigue.

3.2.2 Distance Covered at Different Speed Zones

As mentioned above, the total distance covered by a player during a match or training only shows the total volume performed by the player. The analysis of the distance covered by the player in individual intensity ranges should be much more detailed, but also valuable and interesting for the trainer. These values, presented both in absolute (kilometers or meters) and relative ($m \cdot min^{-1}$), allow for the assessment of the volume performed by the player in each of the analyzed speed zones as well as its intensity. The following arbitrary running speed zones are commonly used in the literature: walking (0.7–7.2 km • h^{-1}), jogging (7.2–14.4 km • h^{-1}), running (14.4–19.8 km • h^{-1}), high-speed running (HSR, 19.8–25.1 km • h^{-1}), and sprinting (>25.2 km • h^{-1}) (Akenhead and Nassis 2016; Beato et al. 2021).

Despite the inherent information available from the distance covered within arbitrary speed zones, this method is biased by the potential players' diversity within a team (e.g., fitness, age, training experience, injury history), consequently masking individual capacities and thus neglecting external load imposed on the individual player. The use of individualized (player-dependent) speed zones has recently therefore been proposed for quantifying external load, reducing the confounding effect of between-player variation in physical capacity (Abbott et al. 2018; Hunter et al. 2014; Mendez-Villanueva et al. 2012).

Regardless of the method of isolating the speed zones (arbitrary or individual), in recent years coaches and analysts have paid more and more attention to the assessment of the distance covered with high and very high intensity by a player during a match or training. It is also related to the fact that with regard to the match running distance, data from the English Premier League between 2006/2007 and 2012/2013 showed a ~ 20% elevation (~3% increase per year) in the distance covered at high-intensity and a ~ 50% increase in the number of high-intensity actions (Barnes et al. 2014). The total sprint distance increased by 8% in the same period. Assuming a comparable trend for the season 2013/2014 and beyond, one would expect an additional increase of >40% in the distance covered at high-intensity running in 2030 compared with that covered during the 2012/2013 season (Nassis et al. 2020).

3.2.3 Accelerations and Decelerations

Accelerations and decelerations are used as another measure of "high-intensity" exertions (Cummins et al. 2013). Players' ability to accelerate and decelerate in soccer is a critical component to their success (Dintiman and Ward 2003). The acceleration and deceleration load in soccer accounts for a significant amount of the metabolic and mechanical stress. Quantifying and managing acceleration and deceleration load is critical to managing the loading stimulus. Acceleration and deceleration counts can be manipulated in training by adjusting training time, drill sizes, and drill numbers. Accelerations and decelerations are reported in meters per second squared ($m{\cdot}s^{-2}$). Accelerations above and decelerations below the configurable threshold for a given analysis system are reported as events. A count of these events is what is reported. Similarly to the work-rate patterns, accelerations and deceleration have also been categorized based upon the speed of the movement, which is thought to represent the "intensity" of the action: low, $<2\ m{\cdot}s^{-2}$; moderate, $2\text{–}4\ m{\cdot}s^{-2}$; and high, $>4\ m{\cdot}s^{-2}$ (Higham et al. 2012).

Derivatives: accelerations per minute or decelerations per minute, total accelerations and decelerations per minute, indicator of the rate of speed change events, accelerations (or decelerations) in speed thresholds.

Given the extremely high energetic demand of accelerating (Osgnach et al. 2010), combined with the disruptive effects on tissue from decelerating (Hewit et al. 2011), it is no surprise that these qualities are likely to be reduced during a match as a result of fatigue (Aughey 2010) – thus potentially reducing the team chances of finally succeeding. Knowing this, sports scientists will often measure the number of accelerations and decelerations their soccer players perform in training or in a match.

3.2.4 Player Load and Accelerometer-Based Metrics

The PlayerLoad indicator is one of the parameters that enables coaches, researchers, and analysts with a limited time to have an insight into the measurement of a player's load. Player load (PL) – (per minute and per meter) is an indicator combining the accelerations produced in three planes of body movement, which were measured here using a triaxial 100-Hz accelerometer incorporated within the GPS devices. Put quite simply, it is the sum of all acceleration forces obtained from the accelerometer data (Weaving et al. 2014), although other accelerometer-based metrics currently exist such as dynamic stress load (Beato et al. 2019). In scientific terms, PlayerLoad or accelerometer-based metrics are an instantaneous rate of change of acceleration divided by a scaling factor. PlayerLoad is measured instantaneously (an athlete's workload at that second) and cumulatively (total workload over a session). Because heel strike force generates vertical accelerations which feed into the formula, PlayerLoad is influenced by distance for players whose team sports (e.g., soccer) involve a significant amount of movement.

Distance and speed metrics are interesting with the appropriate context, but without that context they can be limiting as they do not capture movement and impact. Giving a more complete picture of the workload an athlete gets through, PlayerLoad enables you to personalize and periodize individual athlete loads. If a coach is seeking a quick summary of an athlete's workload, then PlayerLoad is able to provide that.

To avoid bias because of the different durations, these values were normalized for each minute of play. Research on this indicator had reported high intra- and inter-device reliability and it had been shown to be a valid way of monitoring a training load in soccer players (Casamichana and Castellano 2015). For example, PlayerLoad (PL) represented per unit distance covered or time worked is an excellent indicator of movement efficiency. More efficient athletes expose themselves to less PL/min than less efficient ones. Monitoring players over time, variations in this metric are reflective of alterations in movement efficiency, or within a session of intensity of different drills. Validated in many independent research papers, PlayerLoad is an easy-to-use solution for scientifically taking the guesswork out of athlete management and can form a key reference point in your athlete monitoring process.

3.2.5 Metabolic Power

Accelerations and decelerations even at low absolute velocities are high-intensity and energy-demanding activities. However, the way high-intensity activity is determined using velocity thresholds may not account for this (Gaudino et al. 2013). The "metabolic power" is a parameter that aims to provide an overall "estimate" of total internal energy expenditure during a performance based on external load variables. Simply meaning, that if accurate, this metric would enable sports scientists to non-invasively measure the energy expenditure of each athlete during training or competition (Gaudino et al. 2013).

Di Prampero et al. (2005, 2015) developed a mathematical approach to quantify the estimated energy cost associated with any instant change in velocity. It was proposed that accelerated running on a flat terrain is considered energetically equivalent to uphill running at constant speed (Minetti et al. 2002). Metabolic power is calculated as the instant energy cost multiplied by the instant velocity. The ability to calculate instant "energy cost" based on known and measured data and the measurement of "instant velocity" from GPS allows this estimate of metabolic power to be calculated. As both velocity and acceleration are used, it is argued that this provides a better estimation of high-intensity activity. Gaudinho et al. (Gaudino et al. 2013) showed that when the equivalent high-intensity metabolic power threshold (a metabolic power of 20 $W \cdot kg^{-1}$ is considered the equivalent of running at a constant speed of 14.4 $km \cdot h^{-1}$) is used in analysis of soccer training, the actual high-intensity activity could be underestimated by as much as 84 ± 54%. Therefore, the availability of metabolic power calculations through GPS software has been an important parameter in addition to the monitoring of load. Although it was reported above, metabolic power has been heavily criticized by researchers and practitioners (Buchheit et al. 2015; Hader et al. 2016); therefore, further research is needed before completely embracing this training load method.

3.2.6 Conclusions and Practical Applications

Characterized above the internal and external load measures available with today's microtechnology (e.g., GPS) mean that measures from these devices are becoming of increasing interest to scientists and coaches as a noninvasive approach to understand how athletes are coping with training and competition. Knowledge about athletes' responses to the external training load in the training process is crucial in the context of effectively prescribing and monitoring training loads (Akubat et al. 2014). Therefore, it is important to integrate external and internal training load metrics (Burgess 2017). The integrated internal–external load ratio assesses the psychophysiological stress experienced by the athlete (i.e., heart rate, RPE, blood lactate, etc.) during training in the context of the external training load completed and can be used to infer on athlete training status (Bourdon et al. 2017). For example, an increase in the internal load to a standard external load may infer soccer player fatigue or decreased fitness, while a reduced internal load (a lower heart rate or perception of effort to a standard external load) indicates that a player is gaining fitness and coping with training. Furthermore, this may inform on the consequences of training programs (Racinais et al. 2014), identify fatigue during soccer training and competition (Akubat et al. 2014; Kempton et al. 2015), and identify changes in fitness or fatigue status (Buchheit et al. 2013).

All the previously presented assessment methods used during training or a match, training loads, both internal and external, will have their strengths and weaknesses, which often depend on the context of the program to which they are applied and the goals to be achieved. For example, RPE is an inexpensive method that has the advantage of being able to quantify load irrespective of mode or location. In contrast, GPS time–motion analysis is only possible in an outdoor environment without overhead obstructions, requires hardware and software, and is restricted to locomotor movements and position tracking. It is, however, easily interpretable and can be used to prescribe training. Accelerometers, often integrated with other sensors in wearable devices, are similar in cost and hardware and software requirements and have the advantage of being independent of location and activity yet possess limitations in data interpretation and direct use to prescribe training (Bourdon et al. 2017).

Methods that directly quantify a unit of measure (e.g., heart rate, distance, velocity, time) or can count occurrences or repetitions are easily interpretable and can be used to plan and prescribe training, as well as evaluate the demands of competition. The use of composite or derivative methods, typically measured in arbitrary units (e.g., TRIMP derived from heart rate), metabolic power (derived from locomotor acceleration and deceleration), player load (derived from accelerometer acceleration), and RPE (derived from perception of effort), adds more complexity to the interpretation of results but may bring more insight if analyzed correctly (Bourdon et al. 2017).

In summary, the information from this chapter can be used by coaches and analysts in the context of selecting appropriate parameters used to monitor training loads in soccer. Nonetheless, this chapter presents some limitations. For example, we did not characterize the biochemical parameters (creatine kinase, cortisol, testosterone), which are also used quite often as markers assessing the impact of training load. Also, not all sports clubs or coaching staffs have the possibility to evaluate all abovementioned parameters. Regardless of the parameters that we use in our job, it should be remembered that only an adequate standardization of the measurement tools and the ability to draw practical conclusions will allow a reliable assessment of our activities.

References

Abbott W, Brickley G, Smeeton NJ (2018) An individual approach to monitoring locomotive training load in English premier league academy soccer players. Int J Sports Sci Coach 13(3):421–428. https://doi.org/10.1177/1747954118771181

Akenhead R, Nassis GP (2016) Training load and player monitoring in high-level football: current practice and perceptions. Int J Sports Physiol Perform 11(5):587–593. https://doi.org/10.1123/ijspp.2015-0331

Akubat I, Barrett S, Abt G (2014) Integrating the internal and external training loads in soccer. Int J Sports Physiol Perform 9(3):457–462. https://doi.org/10.1123/ijspp.2012-0347

Akubat I, Patel E, Barrett S, Abt G (2012) Methods of monitoring the training and match load and their relationship to changes in fitness in professional youth soccer players. J Sports Sci 30(14):1473–1480. https://doi.org/10.1080/02640414.2012.712711

Alexiou H, Coutts AJ (2008) A comparison of methods used for quantifying internal training load in women soccer players. Int J Sports Physiol Perform 3(3):320–330. https://doi.org/10.1123/ijspp.3.3.320

Andrzejewski M, Chmura P, Konefał M, Kowalczuk E, Chmura J (2018) Match outcome and sprinting activities in match play by elite German soccer players. J Sports Med Phys Fitness 58(6):785. https://doi.org/10.23736/S0022-4707.17.07352-2

Andrzejewski M, Konefał M, Chmura P, Kowalczuk E, Chmura J (2016) Match outcome and distances covered at various speeds in match play by elite German soccer players. Int J Perform Anal Sport 16(3):817–828. https://doi.org/10.1080/24748668.2016.11868930

Andrzejewski M, Pluta B, Konefał M, Konarski J, Chmura J, Chmura P (2019) Activity profile in elite polish soccer players. Res Sports Med 27(4):473–484. https://doi.org/10.1080/15438627.2018.1545648

Aughey RJ (2010) Australian football player work rate: evidence of fatigue and pacing? Int J Sports Physiol Perform 5(3):394–405. https://doi.org/10.1123/ijspp.5.3.394

Aughey RJ (2011) Applications of GPS technologies to field sports. Int J Sports Physiol Perform 6(3):295–310. https://doi.org/10.1123/ijspp.6.3.295

Bangsbo J, Mohr M, Krustrup P (2006) Physical and metabolic demands of training and match-play in the elite football player. J Sports Sci 24(7):665–674. https://doi.org/10.1080/02640410500482529

Banister EW (1991) Modeling elite athletic performance. In: Green JMHWH (ed) Physiological testing of elite athletes. Human Kinetics, Champaign, pp 403–424

Barnes C, Archer D, Hogg B, Bush M, Bradley P (2014) The evolution of physical and technical performance parameters in the English premier league. Int J Sports Med 35(13):1095–1100. https://doi.org/10.1055/s-0034-1375695

Beato M, Coratella G, Stiff A, Dello IA (2018) The validity and between-unit variability of GNSS units (STATSports apex 10 and 18 Hz) for measuring distance and peak speed in team sports. Front Physiol 9:1288. https://doi.org/10.3389/fphys.2018.01288

Beato M, de Keijzer K (2019) The inter-unit and inter-model reliability of GNSS STATSports apex and viper units in measuring peak speed over 5, 10, 15, 20 and 30 meters. Biol Sport 36(4):317–321. https://doi.org/10.5114/biolsport.2019.88754

Beato M, de Keijzer KL, Carty B, Connor M (2019) Monitoring fatigue during intermittent exercise with accelerometer-derived metrics. Front Physiol 10:780. https://doi.org/10.3389/fphys.2019.00780

Beato M, Drust B, Dello IA (2021) Implementing high-speed running and sprinting training in professional soccer. Int J Sports Med 42(4):295–299. https://doi.org/10.1055/a-1302-7968

Beneke R, Leithäuser RM, Ochentel O (2011) Blood lactate diagnostics in exercise testing and training. Int J Sports Physiol Perform 6(1):8–24. https://doi.org/10.1123/ijspp.6.1.8

Borresen J, Ian Lambert M (2009) The quantification of training load, the training response and the effect on performance. Sports Med 39(9):779–795. https://doi.org/10.2165/11317780-000000000-00000

Borresen J, Lambert MI (2008) Quantifying training load: a comparison of subjective and objective methods. Int J Sports Physiol Perform 3(1):16–30. https://doi.org/10.1123/ijspp.3.1.16

Bourdon PC, Cardinale M, Murray A, Gastin P, Kellmann M, Varley MC, Gabbett TJ, Coutts AJ, Burgess DJ, Gregson W, Cable NT (2017) Monitoring athlete training loads: consensus statement. Int J Sports Physiol Perform 12(s2):S2-161-S2-170. https://doi.org/10.1123/IJSPP.2017-0208

Buchheit M, Manouvrier C, Cassirame J, Morin J-B (2015) Monitoring locomotor load in soccer: is metabolic power, powerful? Int J Sports Med 36(14):1149–1155. https://doi.org/10.1055/s-0035-1555927

Buchheit M, Racinais S, Bilsborough JC, Bourdon PC, Voss SC, Hocking J, Cordy J, Mendez-Villanueva A, Coutts AJ (2013) Monitoring fitness, fatigue and running performance during a pre-season training camp in elite football players. J Sci Med Sport 16(6):550–555. https://doi.org/10.1016/j.jsams.2012.12.003

Burgess DJ (2017) The research Doesn't always apply: practical solutions to evidence-based training-load monitoring in elite team sports. Int J Sports Physiol Perform 12(s2):S2-136-S2-141. https://doi.org/10.1123/ijspp.2016-0608

Casamichana D, Castellano J (2015) The relationship between intensity indicators in small-sided soccer games. J Hum Kinet 46(1):119–128. https://doi.org/10.1515/hukin-2015-0040

Chen MJ, Fan X, Moe ST (2002) Criterion-related validity of the Borg ratings of perceived exertion scale in healthy individuals: a meta-analysis. J Sports Sci 20(11):873–899. https://doi.org/10.1080/026404102320761787

Chmura P, Konefał M, Chmura J, Kowalczuk E, Zając T, Rokita A, Andrzejewski M (2018) Match outcome and running performance in different intensity ranges among elite soccer players. Biol Sport 35(2):197–203. https://doi.org/10.5114/biolsport.2018.74196

Chmura P, Konefał M, Wong DP, Figueiredo AJ, Kowalczuk E, Rokita A, Chmura J, Andrzejewski M (2019) Players' physical performance decreased after two-thirds of the season: results of 3 consecutive seasons in the German first Bundesliga. Int J Environ Res Public Health 16(11):2044. https://doi.org/10.3390/ijerph16112044

Chmura P, Liu H, Andrzejewski M, Chmura J, Kowalczuk E, Rokita A, Konefał M (2021) Is there meaningful influence from situational and environmental factors on the physical and technical activity of elite football players? Evidence from the data of 5 consecutive seasons of the German Bundesliga. PLoS One 16(3):e0247771. https://doi.org/10.1371/journal.pone.0247771

Clemente FM, Clark C, Castillo D, Sarmento H, Nikolaidis PT, Rosemann T, Knechtle B (2019) Variations of training load, monotony, and strain and dose-response relationships with maximal aerobic speed, maximal oxygen uptake, and isokinetic strength in professional soccer players. PLoS One 4(12):e0225522. https://doi.org/10.1371/journal.pone.0225522

Cummins C, Orr R, O'Connor H, West C (2013) Global positioning systems (GPS) and microtechnology sensors in team sports: a systematic review. Sports Med 43(10):1025–1042. https://doi.org/10.1007/s40279-013-0069-2

Daanen HAM, Lamberts RP, Kallen VL, Jin A, van Meeteren NLU (2012) A systematic review on heart-rate recovery to monitor changes in training status in athletes. Int J Sports Physiol Perform 7(3):251–260. https://doi.org/10.1123/ijspp.7.3.251

Dellaserra CL, Gao Y, Ransdell L (2014) Use of integrated technology in team sports. J Strength Cond Res 28(2):556–573. https://doi.org/10.1519/JSC.0b013e3182a952fb

di Prampero PE, Atchou G, Brückner JC, Moia C (1986) The energetics of endurance running. Eur J Appl Physiol Occup Physiol 55(3):259–266. https://doi.org/10.1007/BF02343797
di Prampero PE, Botter A, Osgnach C (2015) The energy cost of sprint running and the role of metabolic power in setting top performances. Eur J Appl Physiol 115(3):451–469. https://doi.org/10.1007/s00421-014-3086-4
di Prampero PE, Fusi S, Sepulcri L, Morin JB, Belli A, Antonutto G (2005) Sprint running: a new energetic approach. J Exp Biol 208(14):2809–2816. https://doi.org/10.1242/jeb.01700
Dintiman G, Ward B (2003) Starting and stopping. In: Sports Speed, 3rd edn. Human Kinetics, Champaign, IL, pp 213–217
Edwards S (1993) High performance training and racing. In: The heart rate monitor book. Feet Fleet Press, Carrboro, NC, pp 113–123
Foster C (1998) Monitoring training in athletes with reference to overtraining syndrome. Med Sci Sports Exerc 30(7):1164–1168. https://doi.org/10.1097/00005768-199807000-00023
Foster C, Florhaug JA, Franklin J, Gottschall L, Hrovatin LA, Parker S, Doleshal P, Dodge C (2001) A new approach to monitoring exercise training. J Strength Cond Res 15(1):109–115. https://doi.org/10.1519/00124278-200102000-00019
Gabbett TJ (2016) The training—injury prevention paradox: should athletes be training smarter and harder? Br J Sports Med 50(5):273–280. https://doi.org/10.1136/bjsports-2015-095788
Gabbett TJ, Whyte DG, Hartwig TB, Wescombe H, Naughton GA (2014) The relationship between workloads, physical performance, injury and illness in adolescent male football players. Sports Med 44(7):989–1003. https://doi.org/10.1007/s40279-014-0179-5
Gaudino P, Iaia F, Alberti G, Strudwick A, Atkinson G, Gregson W (2013) Monitoring training in elite soccer players: systematic bias between running speed and metabolic power data. Int J Sports Med 34(11):963–968. https://doi.org/10.1055/s-0033-1337943
Haddad M, Stylianides G, Djaoui L, Dellal A, Chamari K (2017) Session-RPE method for training load monitoring: validity, ecological usefulness, and influencing factors. Front Neurosci 11:612. https://doi.org/10.3389/fnins.2017.00612
Hader K, Mendez-Villanueva A, Palazzi D, Ahmaidi S, Buchheit M (2016) Metabolic power requirement of change of direction speed in young soccer players: not all is what it seems. PLoS One 11(3):e0149839. https://doi.org/10.1371/journal.pone.0149839
Halson SL (2014) Monitoring training load to understand fatigue in athletes. Sports Med 44(S2):139–147. https://doi.org/10.1007/s40279-014-0253-z
Halson SL, Jeukendrup AE (2004) Does overtraining exist? An analysis of overreaching and overtraining research. Sports Med 34(14):967–981. https://doi.org/10.2165/00007256-200434140-00003
Hewit J, Cronin J, Button C, Hume P (2011) Understanding deceleration in sport. Strength Cond J 33(1):47–52. https://doi.org/10.1519/SSC.0b013e3181fbd62c
Higham DG, Pyne DB, Anson JM, Eddy A (2012) Movement patterns in rugby sevens: effects of tournament level, fatigue and substitute players. J Sci Med Sport 15(3):277–282. https://doi.org/10.1016/j.jsams.2011.11.256
Hopkins WG (1991) Quantification of training in competitive sports. Sports Med 12(3):161–183. https://doi.org/10.2165/00007256-199112030-00003
Hunter F, Bray J, Towlson C, Smith M, Barrett S, Madden J, Abt G, Lovell R (2014) Individualisation of time-motion analysis: a method comparison and case report series. Int J Sports Med 36(01):41–48. https://doi.org/10.1055/s-0034-1384547
Iellamo F, Legramante JM, Pigozzi F, Spataro A, Norbiato G, Lucini D, Pagani M (2002) Conversion from vagal to sympathetic predominance with strenuous training in high-performance world class athletes. Circulation 105(23):2719–2724. https://doi.org/10.1161/01.CIR.0000018124.01299.AE
Impellizzeri FM, Marcora SM, Coutts AJ (2019) Internal and external training load: 15 years on. Int J Sports Physiol Perform 14(2):270–273. https://doi.org/10.1123/ijspp.2018-0935
Jaspers A, Brink MS, Probst SGM, Frencken WGP, Helsen WF (2017) Relationships between training load indicators and training outcomes in professional soccer. Sports Med 47(3):533–544. https://doi.org/10.1007/s40279-016-0591-0

Johnston RJ, Watsford ML, Pine MJ, Spurrs RW, Sporri D (2013) Assessment of 5 Hz and 10 Hz GPS units for measuring athlete movement demands. Int J Perform Anal Sport 13(1):262–274. https://doi.org/10.1080/24748668.2013.11868646

Kempton T, Sirotic AC, Coutts AJ (2015) An integrated analysis of match-related fatigue in professional rugby league. J Sports Sci 33(1):39–47. https://doi.org/10.1080/02640414.2014.921832

Konefał M, Chmura P, Tessitore A, Melcer T, Kowalczuk E, Chmura J, Andrzejewski M (2020) The impact of match location and players' physical and technical activities on winning in the German Bundesliga. Front Psychol 11:1748. https://doi.org/10.3389/fpsyg.2020.01748

Konefał M, Chmura P, Zacharko M, Baranowski J, Andrzejewski M, Błażejczyk K, Chmura J (2021) The influence of thermal stress on the physical and technical activities of soccer players: lessons from the 2018 FIFA world cup in Russia. Int J Biometeorol 65(8):1291–1298. https://doi.org/10.1007/s00484-020-01964-3

Little T, Williams AG (2007) Measures of exercise intensity during soccer training drills with professional soccer players. J Strength Cond Res 21(2):367. https://doi.org/10.1519/R-19445.1

Lucia A, Hoyos J, Santalla A, Earnest C, Chicharro J (2003) Tour de France versus Vuelta a ESPA? A: which is harder? Med Sci Sports Exerc 35(5):872–878. https://doi.org/10.1249/01.MSS.0000064999.82036.B4

Martin DT, Andersen MB (2000) Heart rate-perceived exertion relationship during training and taper. J Sports Med Phys Fitness 40(3):201–208

Marynowicz J, Kikut K, Lango M, Horna D, Andrzejewski M (2020) Relationship between the session-RPE and external measures of training load in youth soccer training. J Strength Cond Res 34(10):2800–2804. https://doi.org/10.1519/JSC.0000000000003785

Mendez-Villanueva A, Buchheit M, Simpson B, Bourdon P (2012) Match play intensity distribution in youth soccer. Int J Sports Med 34(02):101–110. https://doi.org/10.1055/s-0032-1306323

Minetti AE, Moia C, Roi GS, Susta D, Ferretti G (2002) Energy cost of walking and running at extreme uphill and downhill slopes. J Appl Physiol 93(3):1039–1046. https://doi.org/10.1152/japplphysiol.01177.2001

Nassis GP, Massey A, Jacobsen P, Brito J, Randers MB, Castagna C, Mohr M, Krustrup P (2020) Elite football of 2030 will not be the same as that of 2020: preparing players, coaches, and support staff for the evolution. Scand J Med Sci Sports 30(6):962–964. https://doi.org/10.1111/sms.13681

Osgnach C, Poser S, Bernardini R, Rinaldo R, di Prampero PE (2010) Energy cost and metabolic power in elite soccer. Med Sci Sports Exerc 42(1):170–178. https://doi.org/10.1249/MSS.0b013e3181ae5cfd

Owen AL, Dunlop G, Rouissi M, Haddad M, Mendes B, Chamari K (2016) Analysis of positional training loads (ratings of perceived exertion) during various-sided games in European professional soccer players. Int J Sports Sci Coach 11(3):374–381. https://doi.org/10.1177/1747954116644064

Plews DJ, Laursen PB, Kilding AE, Buchheit M (2012) Heart rate variability in elite triathletes, is variation in variability the key to effective training? A case comparison. Eur J Appl Physiol 112(11):3729–3741. https://doi.org/10.1007/s00421-012-2354-4

Plews DJ, Laursen PB, Stanley J, Kilding AE, Buchheit M (2013) Training adaptation and heart rate variability in elite endurance athletes: opening the door to effective monitoring. Sports Med 43(9):773–781. https://doi.org/10.1007/s40279-013-0071-8

Portier H, Louisy F, Laude D, Berthelot M, Guézennec CY (2001) Intense endurance training on heart rate and blood pressure variability in runners. Med Sci Sports Exerc 33(7):1120–1125. https://doi.org/10.1097/00005768-200107000-00009

Putlur P, Foster C, Miskowski JA, Kane MK, Burton SE, Scheett TP, McGuigan MR (2004) Alteration of immune function in women collegiate soccer players and college students. J Sports Sci Med 3(4):234–243

Pyne DB, Martin DT (2011) Fatigue-insights from individual and team sports. In: Regulation of fatigue in exercise. Nova Publishers, Hauppauge, NY, pp 177–186

Racinais S, Buchheit M, Bilsborough J, Bourdon PC, Cordy J, Coutts AJ (2014) Physiological and performance responses to a training camp in the heat in professional Australian football players. Int J Sports Physiol Perform 9(4):598–603. https://doi.org/10.1123/ijspp.2013-0284

Reynolds J, Connor M, Jamil M, Beato M (2021) Quantifying and comparing the match demands of U18, U23, and 1ST team English professional soccer players. Front Physiol 12:706451. https://doi.org/10.3389/fphys.2021.706451

Scott TJ, Black CR, Quinn J, Coutts AJ (2013) Validity and reliability of the session-RPE method for quantifying training in Australian football. J Strength Cond Res 27(1):270–276. https://doi.org/10.1519/JSC.0b013e3182541d2e

Shetler K, Marcus R, Froelicher VF, Vora S, Kalisetti D, Prakash M, Do D, Myers J (2001) Heart rate recovery: validation and methodologic issues. J Am Coll Cardiol 38(7):1980–1987. https://doi.org/10.1016/S0735-1097(01)01652-7

Soligard T, Schwellnus M, Alonso J-M, Bahr R, Clarsen B, Dijkstra HP, Gabbett T, Gleeson M, Hägglund M, Hutchinson MR, Janse van Rensburg C, Khan KM, Meeusen R, Orchard JW, Pluim BM, Raftery M, Budgett R, Engebretsen L (2016) How much is too much? (part 1) International Olympic Committee consensus statement on load in sport and risk of injury. Br J Sports Med 50(17):1030–1041. https://doi.org/10.1136/bjsports-2016-096581

Varley MC, Fairweather IH, Aughey RJ (2012) Validity and reliability of GPS for measuring instantaneous velocity during acceleration, deceleration, and constant motion. J Sports Sci 30(2):121–127. https://doi.org/10.1080/02640414.2011.627941

Wallace LK, Slattery KM, Coutts AJ (2009) The ecological validity and application of the session-RPE method for quantifying training loads in swimming. J Strength Cond Res 23(1):33–38. https://doi.org/10.1519/JSC.0b013e3181874512

Wallace LK, Slattery KM, Coutts AJ (2014) A comparison of methods for quantifying training load: relationships between modelled and actual training responses. Eur J Appl Physiol 114(1):11–20. https://doi.org/10.1007/s00421-013-2745-1

Weaving D, Marshall P, Earle K, Nevill A, Abt G (2014) Combining internal- and external-training-load measures in professional Rugby league. Int J Sports Physiol Perform 9(6):905–912. https://doi.org/10.1123/ijspp.2013-0444

Peak Locomotor Demands: Another Approach for Training Load Monitoring

4

José M. Oliva Lozano

Multiple research articles suggest that understanding the match demands is necessary for managing training load in soccer players (Fereday et al. 2020; Martín-Fuentes et al. 2021; Oliva-Lozano et al. 2020, 2021a), especially for teams which compete on leagues with less congested schedules (i.e., one match per week), and therefore, more training days are experienced. Research has provided strength and conditioning coaches with detailed information about the average physical demands of soccer and they can use these data to replicate the external load demands of competition in training situations (Martín-García et al. 2018; Oliva-Lozano et al. 2021a. However, various studies have observed that training drills aimed at replicating average demands might underestimate match demands (Fereday et al. 2020; Oliva-Lozano et al. 2021c).

4.1 Calculation of Peak Locomotor Demands and Practical Implications

Research suggests that it is important to take into account not only the general/average demands but also the peak locomotor demands that the player experiences in specific periods of the match (Oliva-Lozano et al. 2023; Riboli et al. 2021a). These periods are also known as the most demanding passages of play or worst-case scenarios. The periods of peak locomotor demands may have different durations (e.g., 1 or 3 min) and multiple variables (e.g., distance covered, total of high-intensity accelerations or decelerations, etc.) may be used for their calculation (Fereday et al. 2020; Oliva-Lozano et al. 2021c). Overall, the longer the period, the lower the value

J. M. Oliva Lozano (✉)
United States Soccer Federation, Chicago, IL, USA
e-mail: jol908@ual.es

J. M. Oliva Lozano, L. P. Ardigò (eds.), *Training Load in Professional Soccer*,
https://doi.org/10.1007/978-3-031-52087-7_4

the player may achieve (Oliva-Lozano et al. 2021c). In other words, a player may cover ~190 meters per minute given a 1-min phase but a decrease to ~135 meters per minute may be observed in longer passages such as 3-min passages (Oliva-Lozano et al. 2021c). Strength and conditioning coaches use this information to identify the most intense stimulus of match play and design specific drills that replicate match-like intensities in training and return-to-play settings. For instance, training strategies may be designed for a player who is in the latest stages of the return-to-play process through exposure to peak locomotor demands.

Peak locomotor periods may be calculated by different methods (e.g., fixed-length and rolling average methods). For example, if the match has a duration of 90 min and we are using a 1-min period, the fixed-length method registers the demands (e.g., distance covered) minute by minute (e.g., 0′–1′, 130 m; 1′–2′, 140 m; 2′–3′, 150 m; 3′–4′, 160 m, etc.) and selects the minute of the match with the greatest demands (Oliva-Lozano et al. 2021c). However, the rolling averages have shown to be more accurate since these peak periods may happen in very specific time windows (e.g., from 1′35″ to 2′35″ of the match) (Oliva-Lozano et al. 2021c). Previous research examined the interchangeability of both methods for the analysis of peak locomotor periods and the results showed that the use of fixed-length methods significantly underestimated peak demands in all playing positions, so the use of rolling averages was recommended (Fereday et al. 2020; Oliva-Lozano et al. 2021c).

From a practical perspective, one might wonder how frequent these periods of very high intensity occur during the course of the game so that players can have an adequate preparation for such demands. A recent study concluded that significant differences in physical output was observed between the first, second, and third periods of highest locomotor demands in all playing positions and passage durations (Oliva-Lozano et al. 2021d). Nevertheless, the study found that there were some cases (e.g., distance and high-intensity accelerations per minute) in which there were no significant differences between those three peak locomotor periods (Oliva-Lozano et al. 2021d). In consequence, the study suggested that coaches might need to consider not only the physical output in these periods but also the amount of near-to-peak locomotor periods that players may experience in match play.

For this reason, new studies have emerged in this direction and different approaches can be found in the literature. For example, some studies have calculated ranges of percentages of distance covered or high-speed running distance, among other variables, with respect to the 1-min peak values achieved in the match (Oliva-Lozano et al. 2023; Riboli et al. 2021b). Then, the physical output and time spent by the player at different ranges (e.g., distance covered and time require above the 90% of the distance covered in the 1-min peak distance) (Oliva-Lozano et al. 2023; Riboli et al. 2021b). This has very interesting practical applications because if, for example, the high-speed running distance covered by the players is ~50 m in the 1-min peak locomotor demands but the coach knows that matches may require ~6 min above 80% with respect to the 1-min peak locomotor demands that the coach may need to design drills (e.g., transitional games) for this intensity and time window (Oliva-Lozano et al. 2023).

Moreover, coaches need to understand when these periods occur. Another study split the game into periods of 15-min duration: 1′–15′, 15′–30′, 30′–45′, 45′–60′, 60′–75′, and 75′–90′ (Oliva-Lozano et al. 2021b). The locomotor variables were distance covered, sprinting distance above 25.2 km/h, high metabolic load distance above 25.5 W/kg, total of high-intensity accelerations above 3 m/s^2, and high-intensity decelerations below −3 m/s^2. This study found that 0′–15′ was usually the most frequent period of peak locomotor demands (Oliva-Lozano et al. 2021b). However, one of the limitations of this study is that the sample size was not large, and the peak periods were only calculated for 1 min. Research is necessary to identify if longer peak locomotor periods (e.g., 3, 5, or 10 min) also occur in this first period.

4.2 Contextual Factors Related to Match Play Peak Locomotor Demands

A multitude of contextual factors should be considered when examining the variance of periods of peak locomotor demands. The activity profile of any soccer player is multidirectional, multidimensional, and iterative (Martín-García et al. 2018). This chapter provides the reader with a few examples of how context can affect peak locomotor demands.

The greatest peak locomotor demands are usually observed in match day (Oliva-Lozano et al. 2021a). When it comes to training days, MD-4, MD-3, and MD + 1 (for those players in the group that did not play in match day or played significantly less than the rest of players) are the sessions in which the peak locomotor demands of the week are typically registered (Oliva-Lozano et al. 2021a). However, the same study found that the length of the microcycle had a significant effect on the peak locomotor demands in training days' peak periods, but not in match days (Oliva-Lozano et al. 2021a).

Also, research has demonstrated that playing position has a significant effect on the peak locomotor demands (Martín-García et al. 2018; Oliva-Lozano et al. 2020). For example, an investigation observed that central defenders and forwards reported lower peak locomotor demands compared to wide midfielders, fullbacks, and midfielders (Martín-García et al. 2018). Wide midfielders and fullbacks covered greater high metabolic load distance than other positions during all time windows (i.e., 1, 3, 5, and 10 min) (Martín-García et al. 2018).

Furthermore, team formation might be another contextual variable to consider when interpreting peak locomotor demands (Calder and Gabbett 2022; Riboli et al. 2021b). A group of researchers analyzed peak locomotor demands using 4–2–3-1, 3–4-3, and 4–3-3 formations (Calder and Gabbett 2022). Data shows that the 4–3–1-2 yielded greatest accelerations and decelerations for fullbacks and overall distance covered and average speed for forwards (Calder and Gabbett 2022). Another study analyzed 3–4–1-2, 3–4–2-1, 3–5-2, 4–3-3, and 4–4-2, but the authors did not found between-formation differences in high-speed running, sprinting, power metabolic, and high metabolic load distance (Riboli et al. 2021a). However, they found that 1-min peak high-intensity acceleration/deceleration distance was the lowest in 4-4-2 on average and the highest in 4-3-3 for forwards, central, and wide midfielders (Riboli et al. 2021a).

In addition, according to other studies, scoreline and match outcome may be key contextual variables. It has been observed that match outcome had a significant impact on 1-min and 3-min peak locomotor demands while no effect was found for 5-min or 10-min periods (Oliva-Lozano et al. 2020). For example, winning the match yielded greater distance, high-speed running distance, and sprinting distance compared to drawing or losing the match (Oliva-Lozano et al. 2020).

Moreover, one of the greatest studies in this area observed that there might be some physical-tactical trends of professional soccer players during peak 1-min, 3-min, and 5-min periods of match play (Ju et al. 2022). This study analyzed a total of 50 English Premier League matches with 583 player observations (Ju et al. 2022). For instance, this study showed that the largest distances were covered in actions like recovery runs (28–37%) out of possession of the ball and actions related to support play (9–13%) in possession of the ball (Ju et al. 2022). In the following periods, players covered less high-intensity distance compared to the average, being the decline in the next 1-min period more pronounced (Ju et al. 2022).

References

Calder A, Gabbett T (2022) Influence of tactical formation on average and peak demands of elite soccer match-play. IJSC 2(1):1–11. https://doi.org/10.47206/ijsc.v2i1.75

Fereday K, Hills SP, Russell M, Smith J, Cunningham DJ, Shearer D, McNarry M, Kilduff LP (2020) A comparison of rolling averages versus discrete time epochs for assessing the worst-case scenario locomotor demands of professional soccer match-play. J Sci Med Sport 23(8):764–769. https://doi.org/10.1016/j.jsams.2020.01.002

Ju W, Doran D, Hawkins R, Gómez-Díaz A, Martin-Garcia A, Ade JD, Laws A, Evans M, Bradley PS (2022) Contextualised peak periods of play in English premier league matches. Biol Sport 39(4):973–983. https://doi.org/10.5114/biolsport.2022.112083

Martín-Fuentes I, Oliva-Lozano JM, Fortes V, Muyor JM (2021) Effect of playing position, passage duration and starting status on the most demanding passages of match play in professional football. Res Sports Med 25(6):417–426. https://doi.org/10.1080/15438627.2021.1937163

Martín-García A, Casamichana D, Gómez Díaz A, Cos F, Gabbett TJ (2018) Positional differences in the most demanding passages of play in football competition. J Sports Sci Med 17(4):563–570

Oliva-Lozano JM, Fortes V, Muyor JM (2021d) The first, second, and third most demanding passages of play in professional soccer: a longitudinal study. Biol Sport 38(2):165–174. https://doi.org/10.5114/biolsport.2020.97674

Oliva-Lozano JM, Gómez-Carmona CD, Rojas-Valverde D, Fortes V, Pino-Ortega J (2021a) Effect of training day, match, and length of the microcycle on the worst-case scenarios in professional soccer players. Res Sports Med 30(4):425–438. https://doi.org/10.1080/15438627.2021.1895786

Oliva-Lozano JM, Martínez-Puertas H, Fortes V, Muyor JM (2021b) When do soccer players experience the most demanding passages of match play? A longitudinal study in a professional team. Res Sports Med 1–11:101. https://doi.org/10.1080/15438627.2021.1943390

Oliva-Lozano JM, Martín-Fuentes I, Fortes V, Muyor JM (2021c) Differences in worst-case scenarios calculated by fixed length and rolling average methods in professional soccer match-play. Biol Sport 38(3):325–331. https://doi.org/10.5114/biolsport.2021.99706

Oliva-Lozano JM, Riboli A, Fortes V, Muyor JM (2023) Monitoring physical match performance relative to peak locomotor demands: implications for training professional soccer players. Biol Sport 40(2):553–560. https://doi.org/10.5114/biolsport.2023.116450

Oliva-Lozano JM, Rojas-Valverde D, Gómez-Carmona CD, Fortes V, Pino J (2020) Worst case scenario match analysis and contextual variables in professional soccer players: a longitudinal study. Biol Sport 37(4):429–436. https://doi.org/10.5114/biolsport.2020.97067

Riboli A, Esposito F, Coratella G (2021b) The distribution of match activities relative to the maximal intensities in elite soccer players: implications for practice. Res Sports Med 1–12:463. https://doi.org/10.1080/15438627.2021.1895788

Riboli A, Semeria M, Coratella G, Esposito F (2021a) Effect of formation, ball in play and ball possession on peak demands in elite soccer. Biol Sport 38(2):195–205. https://doi.org/10.5114/biolsport.2020.98450

Fatigue in Soccer: Acute and Residual Responses

5

Jeppe F. Vigh-Larsen and Júlio A. Costa

Fatigue in soccer may occur transiently during a game as well as develop progressively, resulting in reduced end-game performance capability, especially in terms of the ability to perform repeated high-intensity exercise. The nature of transient and end-game fatigue development may origin from different sources (e.g., acute perturbations of the intracellular metabolic and ionic environment and/or substantial substrate depletion, muscle damage, changes in core temperature, hydration status, etc.) and may vary significantly between individuals. Moreover, the postgame recovery may be prolonged and involve structural, metabolic, and/or inflammatory/immunological responses and is likely to depend on extrinsic as well as intrinsic factors. Such alterations can be acute following a single game or accumulate during extended periods of fixture congestion or during a long in-season period with a limited amount of periods for rest.

Monitoring sleep and heart rate variability (HRV) in athletes can be useful for early detection and intervention before significant performance and health decrements are observed. Noninvasive and time-efficient methods/equipment such as wearable actigraphy and beat-to-beat HR monitors can provide detailed information about positive and negative adaptions over short and long periods throughout the competitive season. In addition, each athlete can perform the recordings at home, adopting a "real-world scenario" to grant high ecological validity to the research and/or practical interventions. The accumulated knowledge regarding the importance of sleep and HRV (especially during night sleep) has led sleep and HRV monitoring to become a popular strategy among elite athletes, coaches, and supporting staff.

J. F. Vigh-Larsen (✉)
Department of Public Health, Aarhus University, Aarhus, Denmark

J. A. Costa
Portugal Football School, Portuguese Football Federation (FPF), Oeiras, Portugal

J. M. Oliva Lozano, L. P. Ardigò (eds.), *Training Load in Professional Soccer*,
https://doi.org/10.1007/978-3-031-52087-7_5

5.1 Fatigue

The stress associated with training and competition may temporarily impair the physical capacity of a player and result in reduced performance during subsequent games/training sessions as well as increased susceptibility to injury in case of insufficient recovery (Thorpe et al. 2015). This impairment may be acute, lasting minutes or hours, and may stem from metabolic and ionic disturbances and substrate depletion associated with high-intensity exercise (Bangsbo et al. 2006). Moreover, exercise-induced muscle injury and delayed-onset muscle soreness, which often follow training with a high eccentric component, may lead to impairments lasting several days (Thorpe et al. 2015). In addition, perturbations in biochemical markers of inflammatory and immunological variables can persist for prolonged periods of time following match exposure (Ispirlidis et al. 2008). The balance between the stress imposed by training and competition and sufficient recovery is therefore of relevant importance since an imbalance over short durations may result in impaired performance and increased risk of injuries, whereas extended periods of stress/recovery imbalance may result in long-term debilitating effects associated with overreaching and overtraining (Nimmo and Ekblom 2007).

5.1.1 Fatigue during Games

Numerous studies have been published reporting that total distance, and especially distance covered in high-intensity running and sprinting, and the number of explosive accelerations and decelerations, are lower in the second compared to the first half of a match (Vigh-Larsen et al. 2018; Bradley and Noakes 2013; Ingebrigtsen et al. 2015; Andersson et al. 2010; Krustrup et al. 2005; Milanović et al. 2017; Mohr et al. 2003, 2005, 2008). For example, Mohr et al. (2003) reported that the amount of high-intensity running was reduced by 14–45% in the last 15 min compared to the first four 15-min periods of a game. Also, Helgerud et al. (2001) showed that the players who presented higher fatigue levels during the match were those who exhibited a significant decrease in the total number of short passes, as well as in the number of successful short passes, suggesting that impaired technical abilities may be implicated in the fatiguing process. Moreover, the substitute players entering the pitch during the second half of a game has been reported to sprint and run at a markedly higher intensity (63 and 25% more sprint and high-intensity running, respectively) than players who played the entire match (Mohr et al. 2003). These results indicate that performance is attenuated in the second half as a result of fatigue development, which is supported by demonstrations of impaired single and repeated sprint ability as well as reduced neuromuscular function immediately post-game (Rampinini et al. 2011; Ascensão et al. 2008; Krustrup et al. 2006a, 2011; Nybo et al. 2013; Thorlund et al. 2009). Thus, decreases in sprint ability of ~2–7% have been reported (Krustrup et al. 2006a; Rampinini et al. 2011; Ascensão et al. 2008) as well as decreases in maximal voluntary contractions of the knee extensors and flexors of ~9–15% (Rampinini et al. 2011; Ascensão et al. 2008; Krustrup et al. 2011).

5.1.2 End-Game Fatigue

Although muscle fatigue is likely a multifactorial process, the fatigue occurring towards the end of a game has been linked with depletion of the intramuscular stores of carbohydrate (glycogen stores), which is the preferred substrate during soccer match-play (Krustrup et al. 2006a). Accordingly, although muscle glycogen stores appear not to be completely exhausted following a game (reductions from 449 to 255 mmol/kg^{-1} dw), a large proportion of individual slow- and fast-twitch fibers become depleted or nearly depleted of glycogen (Krustrup et al. 2006a). This may result in an inability of a large fraction of fibers to support high-intensity exercise performance as has been demonstrated previously (Balsom et al. 1999). Accordingly, it has been shown that the pre-exercise muscle glycogen status is associated with the amount of total distance and sprint distance covered during a game (Saltin 1973). Moreover, exercise-induced hyperthermia and dehydration has been associated with end-game fatigue development, especially during soccer in the heat, coupled with a marked reduction in high-intensity running (Mohr et al. 2010; Mohr and Krustrup 2013). As such, increases in core temperature to 39.6 °C compared to 38.3 °C during match play in a 43 °C hot environment versus tempered conditions (21 °C) have been shown, which could induce hyperthermia-related central fatigue (Nybo et al. 2013). Likewise, the net fluid loss during that same study was related to impaired repeated sprint performance post-game. In addition, end-game fatigue development has been associated with performance during the yo-yo intermittent recovery test level 1 as the amount of high-intensity running and yo-yo test performance was significantly correlated ($r = 0.51$, Mohr et al. 2010). Thus, a high aerobic capacity may be associated with increased exercise tolerance during the final stages of a game, possibly due to a decreased reliance on anaerobic energy metabolism and subsequent glycogen sparing. The muscle glycogen depletion patterns and role of muscle glycogen for sustained high-intensity exercise performance underline the importance of carbohydrate loading prior to and between games. Moreover, glucose ingestion during games similarly seem to improve performance, possibly through glycogen sparing or alternately by maintenance of blood glucose levels, preventing hypoglycemia-related central fatigue (Baker et al. 2015).

5.1.3 Temporary Fatigue

Evidence of fatigue occurring temporarily after intense periods of a game has been shown in addition to end-game fatigue development. For example, a study performed with male soccer players revealed that the amount of high-intensity running in the 5-min period immediately after the most intense 5-min period recorded during a match was lower than the average of the entire match (Mohr et al. 2003). In support, when players were asked to perform a repeated sprint test immediately after a short-term intense period during the first half, the performance ability was significantly reduced (Krustrup et al. 2006a). Interestingly, when reassessed at half-time following a brief period of recovery, the repeated sprint ability was restored, suggesting that the fatigue occurring during the first half was temporary, whereas after the second half of the game, performance was persistently reduced (Krustrup et al. 2006a). The presence of substantial fatigue occurring transiently during a game highlights the importance of analyzing peak game demands as opposed to tailoring individual fitness regimens based only on total match performance. In this regard, the yo-yo intermittent recovery test level 2 performance has been associated with peak 5-min high-intensity running distance (Krustrup et al. 2006b).

The fatiguing mechanisms underlying temporary fatigue during a game are likely caused by the interactions of several different mechanisms. However, one key factor may be the accumulation of potassium in the muscle interstitium, which may alter the resting membrane potential and muscle excitability (Mohr et al. 2005). In support, the expression of Na^+-K^+ pumps, which role is to protect the resting membrane potential, has been associated with high-intensity performance during games (Mohr et al. 2016). However, other fatiguing mechanisms are likely to contribute to fatigue development during high-intensity exercise, such as increases in reactive oxygen species, creatine phosphate depletion, and accelerated inorganic phosphate and H^+ accumulation, which may alter the muscle calcium kinetics as well as inhibit the contractile machinery and potentially reduce the activity of several key enzymes in muscle metabolism (Allen et al. 2008). However, reduced pH is unlikely to contribute to fatigue in soccer given that muscle pH is only moderately lowered during a game and no relationship with performance impairments has been observed (Mohr et al. 2005).

5.1.4 Post-Match Recovery

Following a single game exposure, fatigue may persist for a prolonged period of time depending on the variable of interest. Accordingly, the fatigue pattern following a soccer game involves multiple mechanisms and responses including neuromuscular alterations, reduced soccer-specific performance, and increased muscle damage, including elevated markers of immunological and inflammatory status, as well as increased muscle soreness and subjective ratings of fatigue (Silva et al. 2018). For example, decreases in neuromuscular function persisting at least until 72 h post-game have been commonly reported (Ispirlidis et al. 2008; Fatouros et al. 2010; Ascensão et al. 2008; Nedelec et al. 2014; Mohr et al. 2015; Draganidis et al. 2015). Also, decreased countermovement jump ability, sprint, and repeated sprint ability may persist for as long as 72 h post-game. Further, markers of muscle damage, including creatine kinase, myoglobin, and lactate dehydrogenase, peak 24–48 h post-game and in some instances remain elevated longer (Silva et al. 2018). Finally, a delayed muscle glycogen resynthesis rate has been reported with only partial resynthesis after 48 h of recovery, especially in type 2 fibers (Gunnarsson et al. 2013; Krustrup et al. 2011). This prolonged recovery of muscle glycogen stores is likely related to the exercise-induced muscle damage response, which may impair the muscle glucose uptake post-exercise (Asp et al. 1995). As a result of this prolonged recovery pattern, the training schedule during the initial 24–48 h of recovery, especially, should be tempered accordingly, in order to avoid excessive loading and increase the risk of injury. In this regard special notice of individual recovery kinetics should be included as discussed below.

5.1.5 Intrinsic and Extrinsic Factors in Fatigue and Recovery

The magnitude of postgame fatigue and the rate of recovery is likely to be associated with intrinsic (age, training status, etc.) as well as extrinsic factors (competition and opposition level, match importance, temperature, etc.) including the individual game requirements (Draganidis et al. 2015; Nedelec et al. 2014; Nybo et al. 2013; Nedelec and Dupont 2019) For example, Draganidis et al. (2015) showed that the reduction in neuromuscular function was higher in the players who covered the largest distances sprinting and accelerating. Similarly, deteriorations in countermovement jump performance has been shown to associate with the number of hard changes in direction and the number of short sprints (<5 m) performed to the increase in muscle soreness (Nedelec et al. 2014). In contrast, soccer played under hypothermic conditions has been shown to accelerate the recovery post-game and attenuate the muscle damage response (creatine kinase), likely due to impaired performance and therefore less high-intensity actions during the actual game (Nybo et al. 2013). Moreover, players with a higher intermittent exercise capacity seem to recover faster following games suggesting that training status may be critical for accelerated postgame recovery kinetics (Draganidis et al. 2015). On this note, large inter-individual variation in post-exercise match recovery patterns has been demonstrated. For example, 0–40% reductions in knee flexor strength has been shown post-game, clearly suggestive of large inter-individual responses (Fransson et al. 2018). Accordingly, it may be critical to monitor individual recovery patterns following each game and/or establish general individual recovery kinetics and adjust the training load accordingly. Moreover, increased resistance to fatigue, for example, through training targeting high-intensity exercise performance capabilities and/or increased neuromuscular function, may reduce the post-game recovery period.

5.1.6 Fixture Congestion

During a regular soccer season the density of games can differ markedly with congested fixtures during specific periods. This may disturb the stress/recovery balance and exacerbate fatigue responses. A study by Mohr et al. (2015) examined the physiological response to a three-game weekly schedule, with 48 h between game 1 and 2 and 72 h between game 2 and 3, and reported strong indications of a larger physiological stress after the middle game which was preceded by the shortest time for recovery. Moreover, Morgans et al. (2014) and Rollo et al. (2014) reported indications of increased physical stress during fixture congestion. Consequently, increased injury susceptibility has been demonstrated highlighting the need for appropriate player rotation and recovery strategies during congested periods (Dupont et al.

2010; Dellal et al. 2015; Bengtsson et al. 2013; Carling et al. 2015). Moreover, mental fatigue has been proposed as an important factor in fatigue development and may be especially relevant when multiple games are played in quick succession (Silva et al. 2018).

5.2 Brief Introduction on Sleep and Heart Rate Variability

The main interest in heart rate variability (HRV) measures is that they are noninvasive, inexpensive, and time-efficient and can be applied routinely and simultaneously in many athletes (i.e., in individual and team sports). While the collection of (beat-by-beat) HRV was initially only possible with expensive laboratory-based electrocardiograph recorders, the recent availability of valid and portable recorders such as HR monitors (Gamelin et al. 2006; Parak and Korhonen 2013; Wallén et al. 2012; Weippert et al. 2010), specifically designed systems (Cassirame et al. 2013; Parrado et al. 2010), or smart phone applications (Flatt and Esco 2013) has substantially boosted the use of HRV monitoring in the field. However, despite its common implementation in the field, HRV monitoring is still not accepted as a gold standard, likely due to the lack of consistency in the literature. While some studies have shown that these measures are sensitive to fitness improvements, fatigue, overload or detraining, others have not (Plews et al. 2013).

Besides the importance of monitoring HRV in athletes, in recent years, growing interest in understanding the sleep of athletes has seen an increase in published studies (Roberts et al. 2019; Walsh et al. 2020). In fact, athletes and coaches have ranked sleep as the most important recovery strategy (Fallon 2007; Walsh et al. 2020). The ability to monitor the sleep duration and quality of sleep obtained by an (elite) athlete may be a useful tool for evaluating recovery from training and competition (Costa et al. 2019a, b, c; Sargent et al. 2016). However, little is known about the sleep characteristics of athletes (Halson 2014; Sargent et al. 2014b). This appears to be a considerable oversight given that sleep has been recognized as an essential component of recovery.

5.2.1 Autonomic Cardiac Function and Sleep Patterns in Soccer

During congested competitive periods, soccer players follow strict match and training schedules which can reduce sleep duration (Sargent et al. 2014a) and impair recovery processes (Fullagar et al. 2016), especially when training sessions and/or matches occur close to bedtime sleep (Fullagar et al. 2016; Vitale et al. 2019).

The effects of physical exercise on sleep have been ascribed to factors such as time of day, chronotype (i.e., an individual's circadian rhythm; Bonato et al. 2017), and training load (Buchheit et al. 2004). Bonato et al. (2017) evaluated whether the time of day (8.00 a.m. vs 8.00 p.m.) and chronotype could influence post-exercise autonomic cardiac control in soccer players in relation to an acute session of high-intensity interval training. The authors showed that circadian typology determined different autonomic responses during recovery from a demanding training bout only in the morning. In a review study, it was suggested that sleep indices were likely dependent on the scheduling of practices of the particular sport (Juliff et al. 2015). The study also stated that 52% of elite athletes subjectively reported sleep disturbances following a late match or training session. Additionally, it was observed that players presented sleep duration within the appropriate healthy range on training and match days concluded before 6 p.m., but slept significantly less with later bedtimes after training sessions and matches starting after 6 p.m. (Fullagar et al. 2016; Nédélec et al. 2019). However, in another study it was found that total sleep time was not affected after performing early evening high-intensity training sessions (starting at ~4.30 p.m. and finishing at 6.30 p.m.) in elite youth soccer players, compared to nights where no evening training was performed (Robey et al. 2014). Other factors could also impair the function of the ANS and sleep, such as travelling, jet lag, and away-match location (Egan-Shuttler et al. 2020).

Nonetheless, it is also important to highlight that sleep patterns and HRV changes that may occur during sleep after physical exercise can be influenced by whether the athletes are exposed to chronic (habitual) or acute (single) late training (Rae et al. 2015) or a night official competition (Vitale et al. 2019). For instance, a recent study showed that sleep duration and quality of female athletes were acutely lower during the night immediately after a night match compared to previous or subsequent nights (Vitale et al. 2019). In addition, another study showed that acute physical exercise (running exercises), in physically active male subjects, caused delayed recovery of nocturnal cardiac autonomic modulation, but no changes in sleep quality (Myllymäki et al. 2012).

For instance, Rae et al. (2015) proposed comparing morning and evening time trial performance, rating of perceived exertion (RPE), and mood states of trained swimmers, considering chronotype and habitual training time of day. The authors found significant diurnal variation in performance when the swimmers were grouped according to habitual training time of day. That is, the swimmers who habitually trained in the morning swam faster at 6.30 a.m. and those who trained in the evening were faster at 6.30 p.m. This suggests that diurnal variation in performance is also related to habitual training time, although it is not clear whether this is due to endogenous factors, training time conditioning, or both.

5.2.1.1 Assessment of Autonomic Cardiac Activity

HRV might provide useful markers of positive and negative adaptations to training and competitions (Halson 2014; Plews et al. 2013). The basic principle of HRV monitoring is to make inferences on possible changes in cardiac autonomic nervous system (ANS) status due to exercise while using repeated HRV measures over time. Since ANS activity is highly sensitive to environmental conditions (e.g., noise, light, temperature; Achten and Jeukendrup 2003), it is important that precautions are taken to standardize recording conditions, in order to isolate the training-induced effects on ANS.

Fluctuations in the R–R (normal-to-normal) intervals may be quantified by numerous techniques, providing indices that reflect the ANS modulation into the heart (Ferreira Jr and Zanesco 2016). With the objective of standardizing the terms and measurement methods in both basic and clinical studies, members of the European Society of Cardiology and the North American Society of Pacing and Electrophysiology created a task force (Heart rate variability. Standards of measurement, physiological interpretation, and clinical use. Task Force of the European Society of Cardiology and the North American Society of Pacing and Electrophysiology 1996). Currently, HRV analysis can be performed using linear methods, which are divided into the time domain and the frequency domain, or using nonlinear methods.

In the linear analysis in the time domain, which is considered as the simplest measure of HRV, the indices are derived from the measurement of intervals between successive normal beats (R–R) in a series of continuous time that can be evaluated by statistical or geometric patterns (Bilchick and Berger 2006; Heart rate variability. Standards of measurement, physiological interpretation, and clinical use. Task Force of the European Society of Cardiology and the North American Society of Pacing and Electrophysiology 1996).

The analysis in the time domain further provides other related measures, which are derived from the difference between the R–R intervals, including the square root of the mean of the sum of the squares of differences between successive R–R intervals (RMSSD), the standard deviation of the R–R intervals (SDNN), the number of pairs of adjacent R–R intervals with a difference of duration longer than 50 ms in the registration period (NN50), and the percentage of successive R–R intervals with a difference of duration longer than 50 ms (pNN50; Ferreira Jr and Zanesco 2016).

These indices are obtained by the difference between successive regular intervals aiming to detect high-frequency oscillations and to provide information on parasympathetic autonomic modulation (Kleiger et al. 2005; Pumprla et al. 2002). Another technique is the Lorenz plot (also known as a Poincaré plot), where each beat is plotted in association with the next beat, providing graphical information and dispersion of the variation in the time series (Ferreira Jr and Zanesco 2016). This analysis can be performed both quantitatively and qualitatively (Billman 2013).

The linear method in the frequency domain (spectral analysis) has been widely used since its introduction in the 1960s as another technique for the investigation of HRV (Ferreira Jr and Zanesco 2016). Unlike the time domain, this technique decomposes the total variability of the signal into specific components that operate in different frequency bands, allowing identification (Shaffer et al. 2014). The calculation of the power of spectral density can be performed through fast Fourier transform techniques or the autoregressive model (Ferreira Jr and Zanesco 2016). As short-time records (2–5 minutes), it is possible to obtain the components of very low frequency (VLF < 0.04 Hz), low frequency (LF; 0.04–0.15 Hz), and high frequency (HF; 0.15–0.4 Hz). In the analysis over 24 h, a fourth peak frequency, represented as ultralow frequency (ULF; 0.003–0.04 Hz), can also be obtained (Billman 2013; Heart rate variability. Standards of measurement, physiological interpretation, and clinical use. Task Force of the European Society of Cardiology and the North American Society of Pacing and Electrophysiology 1996).

The HF component has been widely emphasized as an index that reflects the vagal modulation, whereas the LF component reflects an interaction between sympathetic and parasympathetic activity (Kleiger et al. 2005). On the other hand, experimental data suggest that the rhythm pattern of very low frequency is intrinsically generated by the heart and that its oscillation is modulated by sympathetic nerve endings (McCraty and Shaffer 2015). In addition, the ratio between LF and HF (LF/HF) has been used historically as a measure involving the sympathetic/parasympathetic balance (Pagani et al. 1986). Nevertheless, recent studies suggest that this measure cannot be used as an accurate measure of this balance (Billman 2013).

Evaluation of the HRV from linear methods can be performed from records with durations of 2, 5, and 15 minutes (short time) and over 24 h (long time) (Ferreira Jr and Zanesco 2016). Although it is also used for short-term analysis, the indices obtained in the time domain have been commonly used for long-term records to provide better interpretation of the results, because of the instability of HR over time. Vagal indices of HRV, such as the logarithm of RMSSD (lnRMSSD), reflecting cardiac parasympathetic modulation, are sensitive to fatigue and have been useful in evaluating individual training adaptation in team sports players (Buchheit 2014; de Freitas et al. 2015). Moreover, the weekly (4–7 days) coefficient of variation (CV) of lnRMSSD (lnRMSSDCV) may provide valuable information concerning training-induced perturbations in homeostasis, i.e., can reflect the day-to-day variations in cardiac parasympathetic activity (Buchheit 2014; Flatt and Esco 2015; Nakamura et al. 2020). In general, athletes with a lower lnRMSSDCV are more aerobically fit and seem to cope better with training and match loads (Boullosa et al. 2013; Buchheit et al. 2010; Flatt and Esco 2016). In fact, higher lnRMSSDCV associated with reduced average lnRMSSD during training and matches may be interpreted as a sign of overload (Flatt et al. 2017a, b).

The presence of noise, trends, ectopic beats, and artefacts has been considered as the main problem found in records of HRV. These issues can directly affect the quality of HRV analysis, requiring signal correction (Huikuri et al. 1999). Therefore, ectopic beats are, in general, automatically removed and replaced with interpolated adjacent R–R interval values using a low filter (Tarvainen et al. 2014). In addition, to reduce any potential nonuniformity or skewness in HRV, data can be log-transformed by taking the natural logarithm (Ohlsson et al. 2015) before conducting any statistical analyses (Mourot et al. 2004).

It is also important to note that monitoring training-related cardiac autonomic responses has been facilitated by using after-waking ultrashort-term HRV measurements in male and female athletes (Esco et al. 2016; Fazackerley et al. 2019; Flatt et al. 2017a, b; Stanley et al. 2013). However, in spite of its usefulness, this method does not allow analysis of the time course of post-exercise cardiac autonomic recovery or quantification of HRV during periods of physiological steady state (Al Haddad et al. 2009; Boullosa et al. 2013). In this sense, HRV recordings conducted during night sleep could be an interesting alternative.

HRV data collected during selected slow-wave sleep episodes (SWSE; defined as deep stage of sleep), which offers great signal stability and high standardization of both environmental factors and respiratory influences on HRV, might be preferred (Brandenberger et al. 2005; Buchheit et al. 2004). Nevertheless, night recordings could be difficult to implement daily (Stanley et al. 2013), limiting their usefulness.

The SWSE considers the following:

1. The first 10 min of the first low and regular HR episode lasting at least 15 min.
2. The lowest standard deviation of R–R intervals (SDNN) throughout the period of interest.
3. A circular Poincaré plot (i.e., a round cluster of points in R–R intervals plotted as a function of the previous one).
4. A low inter-beat autocorrelation between successive R–R intervals (i.e., correlation coefficient of the Poincaré plot <0.5).

In summary, monitoring HRV in athletes can be useful for early detection and intervention before significant performance and health decrements are observed. Noninvasive and time-efficient methods/equipment such as wearable beat-to-beat HR monitors can provide detailed information about positive and negative adaptions over short and long periods throughout the competitive season. In addition, each athlete can perform the recordings at home, adopting a "real-world scenario" to grant high ecological validity to the research and/or practical interventions. The accumulated knowledge regarding the importance of HRV has led HRV monitoring to become a popular strategy among elite athletes, coaches, and supporting staff.

5.2.1.2 Assessment of Sleep Patterns

One of the most critical aspects of the recovery continuum for athletes is obtaining enough sleep duration and quality of sleep. It is recommended that adults sleep at least 7 h per night and achieve a sleep efficiency (i.e., time asleep as a percentage of time in bed) of at least $\geq 75\%$ on a regular basis to promote health (Ohayon et al. 2017; Watson et al. 2015). However, athletes usually sleep less than 7 h (Gupta et al. 2017), requiring more accumulated time to sleep. In fact, extended sleep duration can lead to better psychomotor accomplishment and technical accuracy (Mah et al. 2011), with likely positive effects on competitive performance (Kölling et al. 2016a, b). Interestingly, most of the research examining athletes' sleep has been derived only from subjective tools (e.g., diaries; Knufinke et al. 2018). This is a problem because subjective tools, while useful for monitoring large cohorts, typically correlate poorly with objective data (Dunican et al. 2017). To detect and manage sleep disturbances, it is important to monitor habits and perceptions of sleep with subjective and objective measures (Myllymäki et al. 2011). Overall, two methods are primarily utilized to assess sleep: PSG and actigraphy (Nédélec et al. 2015).

PSG is considered by many to be the gold standard for measuring sleep and typically includes an assessment of eye movement, brain activity, HR, muscle activity, oxygen saturation, breathing rate, and body movement (Roomkham et al. 2018). PSG allows for the determination of sleep stages (rapid eye movement and non-rapid eye movement). PSG is typically only utilized to assess specific sleep disorders as it is an expensive, obtrusive, and complex technique, requiring expertise in setting up the individual to be monitored and manually scoring the sleep data. Further, PSG typically occurs in a laboratory and therefore is impractical for longitudinal monitoring. Finally, PSG may be useful in a research context where understanding the effects of an intervention on sleep staging may be of interest.

Actigraphy is usually measured by a small wrist device worn on the nondominant arm (Sargent et al. 2016). According to Gögenur (2010), wrist movements are continuously translated into an electronic signal through the displacement of a piezoelectric transducer. Thereby, the signal is recorded when movement occurs in all three dimensions and thus distinguishes between "motionless/resting" and "lying" (Peterson et al. 2012). Activity counts are then provided on a minute-by-minute basis, for example, by the so-called zero-crossing mode (Gögenur et al. 2009a, b). In the zero-crossing mode, the number of times per minute where the activity crosses zero activity is registered (Gögenur 2010). These data are then downloaded to a software where the final data analysis is performed. Additionally, data collection starts only when the device is worn on the body and terminates autonomously when off the body (Kölling et al. 2016a, b).

Various actigraphic devices have already been applied in sports settings to monitor sleep parameters (Fietze et al. 2009; Hausswirth et al. 2014; Mah et al. 2011). Several studies have assessed the validity of activity monitors for measuring sleep by comparing sleep/wake durations determined by PSG with sleep/wake durations determined by activity monitors. In healthy adults, high correlations have been reported for sleep duration (i.e., 0.89–0.98; de Souza et al. 2003; Kripke et al. 1978; Signal et al. 2005) and moderate-to-high correlations have been reported for wake time within sleep (i.e., 0.36–0.85; de Souza et al. 2003; Kripke et al. 1978; Mullaney et al. 1980). More recently, validation of activity monitors has moved beyond comparing sleep/wake durations towards considering epoch-for-epoch matches with PSG. Agreement between PSG and activity monitors is high, with rates ranging from 77% to 91% (Kosmadopoulos et al. 2014; Paquet et al. 2007; Signal et al. 2005).

Overall, wrist-worn accelerometers allow estimation of total sleep time (total amount of sleep obtained), time in bed (time between lying down until getting up the next day), wake up time (time between the last minute of sleep and getting up from bed), sleep onset time (time of the first epoch of sleep between time of trying to initiate sleep and time at wake up), wake after sleep onset (number of min awake after sleep onset), sleep fragmentation index (sum of mobility and immobility accesses in one minute, divided by the number of immobility accesses), latency (time in minutes attempting to fall asleep), and sleep efficiency (percentage of time in bed that was spent asleep; Sargent et al. 2016). However, activity monitors tend to underestimate sleep in people who exhibit high levels of movement during light sleep (Tryon 2004). This raises a potential issue with the use of activity monitors for measuring sleep in (elite) athletes.

Several studies indicate that elite athletes obtain less sleep than the general population (Roach et al. 2013; Sargent et al. 2014b) and/or exhibit greater movement and fragmentation during sleep (Leeder et al. 2012; Taylor et al. 1997). Given the sleep characteristics of elite athletes, it is important to establish how well activity monitors detect sleep and wake variables in this population.

Finally, subjective ratings can be obtained via sleep logs, which provide useful information about the individual's habits and perception of sleep (Baker et al. 1999). Nevertheless, subjective reports might deviate from objective measures (Kawada 2008), especially with regard to mood and memory biases, while personality characteristics may also affect self-reported sleep ratings (Jackowska et al. 2011). Indeed, some discrepancies have been detected when comparing subjective parameters with objective measures (Kölling et al. 2016a, 2016b).

5.2.2 Recovery Strategies: Sleep Hygiene

In soccer, sleep impairment may be acutely dictated by some constraints, such as playing or training at night close to bedtime, congested scheduling, travelling, light exposure, use of products containing caffeine or alcohol in the period preceding bedtime, and variations in wake-up time or bedtime (Nédélec et al. 2015; Walsh et al. 2020). Thus, proper sleep hygiene is important for all athletes, including sleep environment and sleep scheduling. Sleep environments should be comfortable, cool, dark, without electronic devices, and with minimal ambient noise or distraction (Watson 2017; Walsh et al. 2020). To the extent that training and competition schedules allow, athletes should be encouraged to establish consistent sleep and wake times and incorporate a 30- to 60-min period of quiet relaxation before bedtime that can help facilitate sleep onset (Watson 2017; Walsh et al. 2020). Efforts should be made to limit the effects of training and competition on sleep schedules to reduce the risk of sleep restriction in athletes. Variation in training times should be minimized and early morning and late evening training and competitions should be avoided (Nédélec et al. 2015).

One possible way to examine the effect of sleep on performance is to extend the amount of sleep an athlete receives and determine the effects on subsequent performance. For instance, Mah et al. (2011) instructed six basketball players to obtain as much extra sleep as possible following 2 weeks of normal sleep habits. Faster sprint times and increased free-throw accuracy were observed at the end of the sleep extension period. Mood was also significantly improved, with increased vigor and decreased fatigue (Mah et al. 2011). Thus, and according to the data from this study, Mah et al. (2011) suggested that increasing the amount of sleep an athlete receives may significantly enhance performance.

Athletes suffering from some degree of sleep loss may also benefit from a brief nap, particularly if a training session is to be performed in the afternoon or evening. Waterhouse et al. (2007) investigated the effects of a lunchtime nap on sprint performance following partial sleep deprivation (4 h of sleep). Following a 30-min nap, 20-m sprint performance was increased (compared to no nap), alertness was increased, and sleepiness was decreased. In terms of cognitive performance, sleep supplementation in the form of napping has been shown to have a positive influence on cognitive tasks (Postolache et al. 2005). Naps can markedly reduce sleepiness and can be beneficial when learning skills, strategy, or tactics are demanded in sleep-deprived individuals (Postolache et al. 2005). Napping may be beneficial for athletes who have to routinely wake up early for training or competition and for athletes who are experiencing sleep deprivation (Waterhouse et al. 2007). Furthermore, naps may provide an additional performance benefit during periods of unavoidable sleep restriction (Brooks and Lack 2006). Naps should be relatively brief (~30 min) to prevent sleep inertia and avoided late in the day to prevent any disruption of nighttime sleep (Walsh et al. 2020; Watson 2017). While further research is needed to clarify the role of naps in athletic performance, the available evidence suggests that naps could be a useful way to increase total sleep duration during periods when sleep restriction is unavoidable, but not necessarily as a substitute for nighttime sleep.

It is important to highlight that other types of sleep hygiene strategies exist, especially used in elite soccer players, such as red-light therapy (body receiving irradiation from a red-light therapy instrument), relaxation and brainwave entrainment (involves stimulating the brain during sleep with frequencies between 1 and 9 Hz in a sequence mimicking the healthy human sleep cycle), and sleep medication (includes hypnotics, medium half-life benzodiazepines [e.g., temazepam], and short half-life non-benzodiazepine medications [e.g., zolpidem]). These medications do not contravene the World Anti-Doping Agency rules (Nédélec et al. 2015).

In summary, sleep is extremely important for numerous biological functions and sleep deprivation can have significant effects on athletic performance, especially sub-maximal, prolonged exercise. From the available evidence, it appears that athletes may be obtaining less than 8 h of sleep per night and that increasing sleep (sleep extension) or napping may be useful to increase the total number of hours of sleep and thereby enhance performance.

References

Achten J, Jeukendrup AE (2003) Heart rate monitoring: applications and limitations. Sports Med 33(7):517–538. https://doi.org/10.2165/00007256-200333070-00004

Al Haddad H, Laursen PB, Ahmaidi S, Buchheit M (2009) Nocturnal heart rate variability following supramaximal intermittent exercise. Int J Sports Physiol Perform 4(4):435–447. https://doi.org/10.1123/ijspp.4.4.435

Allen DG, Lamb GD, Westerblad H (2008) Skeletal muscle fatigue: cellular mechanisms. Physiol Rev 88(1):287–332. https://doi.org/10.1152/physrev.00015.2007

Andersson HA, Randers MB, Heiner-Møller A, Krustrup P, Mohr M (2010) Elite female soccer players perform more high-intensity running when playing in international games compared with domestic league games. J Strength Cond Res 24(4):912–919. https://doi.org/10.1519/JSC.0b013e3181d09f21

Anon (1996) Heart rate variability. Standards of measurement, physiological interpretation, and clinical use. Task force of the European Society of Cardiology and the north American Society of Pacing and Electrophysiology. Eur Heart J 17(3):354–381

Ascensão A, Rebelo A, Oliveira E, Marques F, Pereira L, Magalhães J (2008) Biochemical impact of a soccer match - analysis of oxidative stress and muscle damage markers throughout recovery. Clin Biochem 41(10–11):841–851. https://doi.org/10.1016/j.clinbiochem.2008.04.008

Asp S, Daugaard JR, Richter EA (1995) Eccentric exercise decreases glucose transporter GLUT4 protein in human skeletal muscle. J Physiol 482(Pt3):705–712. https://doi.org/10.1113/jphysiol.1995.sp020553

Baker FC, Maloney S, Driver HS (1999) A comparison of subjective estimates of sleep with objective polysomnographic data in healthy men and women. J Psychosom Res 47(4):335–341. https://doi.org/10.1016/s0022-3999(99)00017-3

Baker LB, Rollo I, Stein KW, Jeukendrup AE (2015) Acute effects of carbohydrate supplementation on intermittent sports performance. Nutrients 7(7):5733–5763. https://doi.org/10.3390/nu7075249

Balsom PD, Gaitanos GC, Soderlund K, Ekblom B (1999) High-intensity exercise and muscle glycogen availability in humans. Acta Physiol Scand 165(4):337–345. https://doi.org/10.1046/j.1365-201x.1999.00517.x

Bangsbo J, Mohr M, Krustrup P (2006) Physical and metabolic demands of training and match-play in the elite football player. J Sports Sci 24(7):665–674. https://doi.org/10.1080/02640410500482529

Bengtsson H, Ekstrand J, Hagglund M (2013) Muscle injury rates in professional football increase with fixture congestion: an 11-year follow-up of the UEFA champions league injury study. Br J Sports Med 47(12):743–747. https://doi.org/10.1136/bjsports-2013-092383

Bilchick KC, Berger RD (2006) Heart rate variability. J Cardiovasc Electrophysiol 17(6):691–694. https://doi.org/10.1111/j.1540-8167.2006.00501.x

Billman GE (2013) The LF/HF ratio does not accurately measure cardiac sympatho-vagal balance. Front Physiol 4:26. https://doi.org/10.3389/fphys.2013.00026

Bonato M, Agnello L, Galasso L, Montaruli A, Roveda E, Merati G, La Torre A, Vitale JA (2017) Acute modification of cardiac autonomic function of high-intensity interval training in collegiate male soccer players with different chronotype: a cross-over study. J Sports Sci Med 16(2):286–294

Boullosa DA, Abreu L, Nakamura FY, Muñoz VE, Domínguez E, Leicht AS (2013) Cardiac autonomic adaptations in elite Spanish soccer players during preseason. Int J Sports Physiol Perform 8(4):400–409. https://doi.org/10.1123/ijspp.8.4.400

Bradley PS, Noakes TD (2013) Match running performance fluctuations in elite soccer: indicative of fatigue, pacing or situational influences? J Sports Sci 31(15):1627–1638. https://doi.org/10.1080/02640414.2013.796062

Brandenberger G, Buchheit M, Ehrhart J, Simon C, Piquard F (2005) Is slow wave sleep an appropriate recording condition for heart rate variability analysis? Auton Neurosci 121(1–2):81–86. https://doi.org/10.1016/j.autneu.2005.06.002

Brooks A, Lack L (2006) A brief afternoon nap following nocturnal sleep restriction: which nap duration is most recuperative? Sleep 29(6):831–840. https://doi.org/10.1093/sleep/29.6.831

Buchheit M (2014) Monitoring training status with HR measures: do all roads lead to Rome? Front Physiol 5:73. https://doi.org/10.3389/fphys.2014.00073

Buchheit M, Mendez-Villanueva A, Quod MJ, Poulos N, Bourdon P (2010) Determinants of the variability of heart rate measures during a competitive period in young soccer players. Eur J Appl Physiol 109(5):869–878. https://doi.org/10.1007/s00421-010-1422-x

Buchheit M, Simon C, Piquard F, Ehrhart J, Brandenberger G (2004) Effects of increased training load on vagal-related indexes of heart rate variability: a novel sleep approach. Am J Physiol Heart Circ Physiol 287(6):H2813–H2818. https://doi.org/10.1152/ajpheart.00490.2004

Carling C, McCall A, Le Gall F, Dupont G (2015) The impact of short periods of match congestion on injury risk and patterns in an elite football club. Br J Sports Med 50:764. https://doi.org/10.1136/bjsports-2015-095501

Cassirame J, Stuckey MI, Sheppard F, Tordi N (2013) Accuracy of the Minicardio system for heart rate variability analysis compared to ECG. J Sports Med Phys Fitness 53(3):248–254

Costa JA, Brito J, Nakamura FY, Figueiredo P, Oliveira E, Rebelo A (2019a) Sleep patterns and nocturnal cardiac autonomic activity in female athletes are affected by the timing of exercise and match location. Chronobiol Int 36(3):360–373. https://doi.org/10.1080/07420528.2018.1545782

Costa JA, Brito J, Nakamura FY, Oliveira EM, Costa OP, Rebelo AN (2019c) Does night training load affect sleep patterns and nocturnal cardiac autonomic activity in high-level female soccer players? Int J Sports Physiol Perform 14(6):779–787. https://doi.org/10.1123/ijspp.2018-0652

Costa J, Figueiredo P, Nakamura F, Rago V, Rebelo A, Brito J (2019b) Intra-individual variability of sleep and nocturnal cardiac autonomic activity in elite female soccer players during an international tournament. PLoS One 14(9):e0218635. https://doi.org/10.1371/journal.pone.0218635

de Freitas VH, Pereira LA, de Souza EA, Leicht AS, Bertollo M, Nakamura FY (2015) Sensitivity of the Yo-Yo intermittent recovery test and cardiac autonomic responses to training in futsal players. Int J Sports Physiol Perform 10(5):553–558. https://doi.org/10.1123/ijspp.2014-0365

de Souza L, Benedito-Silva AA, Pires ML, Poyares D, Tufik S, Calil HM (2003) Further validation of actigraphy for sleep studies. Sleep 26(1):81–85. https://doi.org/10.1093/sleep/26.1.81

Dellal A, Lago-Penas C, Rey E, Chamari K, Orhant E (2015) The effects of a congested fixture period on physical performance, technical activity and injury rate during matches in a professional soccer team. Br J Sports Med 49(6):390–394. https://doi.org/10.1136/bjsports-2012-091290

Draganidis D, Chatzinikolaou A, Avloniti A, Barbero-Alvarez JC, Mohr M, Malliou P, Gourgoulis V, Deli CK, Douroudos II, Margonis K, Gioftsidou A, Flouris AD, Jamurtas AZ, Koutedakis Y, Fatouros IG (2015) Recovery kinetics of knee flexor and extensor strength after a football match. PLoS One 10(6):e0128072. https://doi.org/10.1371/journal.pone.0128072

Dunican IC, Martin DT, Halson SL, Reale RJ, Dawson BT, Caldwell JA, Jones MJ, Eastwood PR (2017) The effects of the removal of electronic devices for 48 hours on sleep in elite judo athletes. J Strength Cond Res 31(10):2832–2839. https://doi.org/10.1519/JSC.0000000000001697

Dupont G, Nedelec M, McCall A, McCormack D, Berthoin S, Wisloff U (2010) Effect of 2 soccer matches in a week on physical performance and injury rate. Am J Sports Med 38(9):1752–1758. https://doi.org/10.1177/0363546510361236

Egan-Shuttler JD, Edmonds R, Ives SJ (2020) The efficacy of heart rate variability in tracking travel and training stress in youth female rowers: a preliminary study. J Strength Cond Res 34(11):3293–3300. https://doi.org/10.1519/JSC.0000000000002499

Esco MR, Flatt AA, Nakamura FY (2016) Initial weekly HRV response is related to the prospective change in VO2max in female soccer players. Int J Sports Med 37(6):436–441. https://doi.org/10.1055/s-0035-1569342

Fallon KE (2007) Blood tests in tired elite athletes: expectations of athletes, coaches and sport science/sports medicine staff. Br J Sports Med 41(1):41–44. https://doi.org/10.1136/bjsm.2006.030999

Fatouros IG, Chatzinikolaou A, Douroudos II, Nikolaidis MG, Kyparos A, Margonis K, Michailidis Y, Vantarakis A, Taxildaris K, Katrabasas I, Mandalidis D, Kouretas D, Jamurtas AZ (2010) Time-course of changes in oxidative stress and antioxidant status responses following a soccer game. J Strength Cond Res 24(12):3278–3286. https://doi.org/10.1519/JSC.0b013e3181b60444

Fazackerley LA, Fell JW, Kitic CM (2019) The effect of an ultra-endurance running race on heart rate variability. Eur J Appl Physiol 119(9):2001–2009. https://doi.org/10.1007/s00421-019-04187-6

Ferreira M Jr, Zanesco A (2016) Heart rate variability as important approach for assessment autonomic modulation. Mot Rev Educ Fís 22(2):3–8. https://doi.org/10.1590/S1980-65742016000200001

Fietze I, Strauch J, Holzhausen M, Glos M, Theobald C, Lehnkering H, Penzel T (2009) Sleep quality in professional ballet dancers. Chronobiol Int 26(6):1249–1262. https://doi.org/10.3109/07420520903221319

Flatt AA, Esco MR (2013) Validity of the ithlete™ smart phone application for determining ultra-short-term heart rate variability. J Hum Kinet 39:85–92. https://doi.org/10.2478/hukin-2013-0071

Flatt AA, Esco MR (2015) Smartphone-derived heart-rate variability and training load in a Women's soccer team. Int J Sports Physiol Perform 10(8):994–1000. https://doi.org/10.1123/ijspp.2014-0556
Flatt AA, Esco MR (2016) Evaluating individual training adaptation with smartphone-derived heart rate variability in a collegiate female soccer team. J Strength Cond Res 30(2):378–385. https://doi.org/10.1519/JSC.0000000000001095
Flatt AA, Esco MR, Nakamura FY (2017b) Individual heart rate variability responses to preseason training in high level female soccer players. J Strength Cond Res 31(2):531–538. https://doi.org/10.1519/JSC.0000000000001482
Flatt AA, Esco MR, Nakamura FY, Plews DJ (2017a) Interpreting daily heart rate variability changes in collegiate female soccer players. J Sports Med Phys Fitness 57(6):907–915. https://doi.org/10.23736/S0022-4707.16.06322-2
Fransson D, Vigh-Larsen JF, Fatouros IG, Krustrup P, Mohr M (2018) Fatigue responses in various muscle groups in well-trained competitive male players after a simulated soccer game. J Hum Kinet 61:85–97. https://doi.org/10.1515/hukin-2017-0129
Fullagar HH, Skorski S, Duffield R, Julian R, Bartlett J, Meyer T (2016) Impaired sleep and recovery after night matches in elite football players. J Sports Sci 34(14):1333–1339. https://doi.org/10.1080/02640414.2015.1135249
Gamelin FX, Berthoin S, Bosquet L (2006) Validity of the polar S810 heart rate monitor to measure R-R intervals at rest. Med Sci Sports Exerc 38(5):887–893. https://doi.org/10.1249/01.mss.0000218135.79476.9c
Gögenur I (2010) Postoperative circadian disturbances. Dan Med Bull 57(12):B4205
Gögenur I, Bisgaard T, Burgdorf S, van Someren E, Rosenberg J (2009a) Disturbances in the circadian pattern of activity and sleep after laparoscopic versus open abdominal surgery. Surg Endosc 23(5):1026–1031. https://doi.org/10.1007/s00464-008-0112-9
Gögenur I, Kücükakin B, Bisgaard T, Kristiansen V, Hjortsø NC, Skene DJ, Rosenberg J (2009b) The effect of melatonin on sleep quality after laparoscopic cholecystectomy: a randomized, placebo-controlled trial. Anesth Analg 108(4):1152–1156. https://doi.org/10.1213/ane.0b013e31819a6cf0
Gunnarsson TP, Bendiksen M, Bischoff R, Christensen PM, Lesivig B, Madsen K, Stephens F, Greenhaff P, Krustrup P, Bangsbo J (2013) Effect of whey protein- and carbohydrate-enriched diet on glycogen resynthesis during the first 48 h after a soccer game. Scand J Med Sci Sports 23(4):508–515. https://doi.org/10.1111/j.1600-0838.2011.01418.x
Gupta L, Morgan K, Gilchrist S (2017) Does elite sport degrade sleep quality? A systematic review. Sports Med 47(7):1317–1333. https://doi.org/10.1007/s40279-016-0650-6
Halson SL (2014) Sleep in elite athletes and nutritional interventions to enhance sleep. Sports Med 44(Suppl 1 (Suppl 1)):S13–S23. https://doi.org/10.1007/s40279-014-0147-0
Hausswirth C, Louis J, Aubry A, Bonnet G, Duffield R, Meur LE, Y. (2014) Evidence of disturbed sleep and increased illness in overreached endurance athletes. Med Sci Sports Exerc 46(5):1036–1045. https://doi.org/10.1249/MSS.0000000000000177
Helgerud J, Engen LC, Wisloff U, Hoff J (2001) Aerobic endurance training improves soccer performance. Med Sci Sports Exerc 33(11):1925–1931. https://doi.org/10.1097/00005768-200111000-00019
Huikuri HV, Mäkikallio T, Airaksinen KE, Mitrani R, Castellanos A, Myerburg RJ (1999) Measurement of heart rate variability: a clinical tool or a research toy? J Am Coll Cardiol 34(7):1878–1883. https://doi.org/10.1016/s0735-1097(99)00468-4
Ingebrigtsen J, Dalen T, Hjelde GH, Drust B, Wisløff U (2015) Acceleration and sprint profiles of a professional elite football team in match play. Eur J Sport Sci 15(2):101–110. https://doi.org/10.1080/17461391.2014.933879
Ispirlidis I, Fatouros IG, Jamurtas AZ, Nikolaidis MG, Michailidis I, Douroudos I, Margonis K, Chatzinikolaou A, Kalistratos E, Katrabasas I, Alexiou V, Taxildaris K (2008) Time-course of changes in inflammatory and performance responses following a soccer game. Clin J Sport Med 18(5):423–431. https://doi.org/10.1097/JSM.0b013e3181818e0b

Jackowska M, Dockray S, Hendrickx H, Steptoe A (2011) Psychosocial factors and sleep efficiency: discrepancies between subjective and objective evaluations of sleep. Psychosom Med 73(9):810–816. https://doi.org/10.1097/PSY.0b013e3182359e77

Juliff LE, Halson SL, Peiffer JJ (2015) Understanding sleep disturbance in athletes prior to important competitions. J Sci Med Sport 18(1):13–18. https://doi.org/10.1016/j.jsams.2014.02.007

Kawada T (2008) Agreement rates for sleep/wake judgments obtained via accelerometer and sleep diary: a comparison. Behav Res Methods 40(4):1026–1029. https://doi.org/10.3758/BRM.40.4.1026

Kleiger RE, Stein PK, Bigger JT Jr (2005) Heart rate variability: measurement and clinical utility. Ann Noninvasive Electrocardiol 10(1):88–101. https://doi.org/10.1111/j.1542-474X.2005.10101.x

Knufinke M, Nieuwenhuys A, Geurts S, Coenen A, Kompier M (2018) Self-reported sleep quantity, quality and sleep hygiene in elite athletes. J Sleep Res 27(1):78–85. https://doi.org/10.1111/jsr.12509

Kölling S, Endler S, Ferrauti A, Meyer T, Kellmann M (2016a) Comparing subjective with objective sleep parameters via multisensory Actigraphy in German physical education students. Behav Sleep Med 14(4):389–405. https://doi.org/10.1080/15402002.2015.1017096

Kölling S, Steinacker JM, Endler S, Ferrauti A, Meyer T, Kellmann M (2016b) The longer the better: sleep-wake patterns during preparation of the world rowing junior championships. Chronobiol Int 33(1):73–84. https://doi.org/10.3109/07420528.2015.1118384

Kosmadopoulos A, Sargent C, Darwent D, Zhou X, Roach GD (2014) Alternatives to polysomnography (PSG): a validation of wrist actigraphy and a partial-PSG system. Behav Res Methods 46(4):1032–1041. https://doi.org/10.3758/s13428-013-0438-7

Kripke DF, Mullaney DJ, Messin S, Wyborney VG (1978) Wrist actigraphic measures of sleep and rhythms. Electroencephalogr Clin Neurophysiol 44(5):674–676. https://doi.org/10.1016/0013-4694(78)90133-5

Krustrup P, Mohr M, Ellingsgaard H, Bangsbo J (2005) Physical demands during an elite female soccer game: importance of training status. Med Sci Sports Exerc 37(7):1242–1248. https://doi.org/10.1249/01.mss.0000170062.73981.94

Krustrup P, Mohr M, Nybo L, Jensen JM, Nielsen JJ, Bangsbo J (2006b) The Yo-Yo IR2 test: physiological response, reliability, and application to elite soccer. Med Sci Sports Exerc 38(9):1666–1673. https://doi.org/10.1249/01.mss.0000227538.20799.08

Krustrup P, Mohr M, Steensberg A, Bencke J, Kjaer M, Bangsbo J (2006a) Muscle and blood metabolites during a soccer game: implications for sprint performance. Med Sci Sports Exerc 38(6):1165–1174. https://doi.org/10.1249/01.mss.0000222845.89262.cd

Krustrup P, Ørtenblad N, Nielsen J, Nybo L, Gunnarsson TP, Iaia FM, Madsen K, Stephens F, Greenhaff P, Bangsbo J (2011) Maximal voluntary contraction force, SR function and glycogen resynthesis during the first 72 h after a high-level competitive soccer game. Eur J Appl Physiol 111(12):2987–2995. https://doi.org/10.1007/s00421-011-1919-y

Leeder J, Glaister M, Pizzoferro K, Dawson J, Pedlar C (2012) Sleep duration and quality in elite athletes measured using wristwatch actigraphy. J Sports Sci 30(6):541–545. https://doi.org/10.1080/02640414.2012.660188

Mah CD, Mah KE, Kezirian EJ, Dement WC (2011) The effects of sleep extension on the athletic performance of collegiate basketball players. Sleep 34(7):943–950. https://doi.org/10.5665/SLEEP.1132

McCraty R, Shaffer F (2015) Heart rate variability: new perspectives on physiological mechanisms, assessment of self-regulatory capacity, and health risk. Glob Adv Health Med 4(1):46–61. https://doi.org/10.7453/gahmj.2014.073

Milanović Z, Sporiš G, James N, Trajković N, Ignjatović A, Sarmento H, Trecroci A, Mendes B (2017) Physiological demands, morphological characteristics, physical abilities and injuries of female soccer players. J Hum Kinet 60:77–83. https://doi.org/10.1515/hukin-2017-0091

Mohr M, Draganidis D, Chatzinikolaou A, Barbero-Alvarez JC, Castagna C, Douroudos I, Avloniti A, Margeli A, Papassotiriou I, Flouris AD, Jamurtas AZ, Krustrup P, Fatouros IG (2015)

Muscle damage, inflammatory, immune and performance responses to three football games in 1 week in competitive male players. Eur J Appl Physiol 116:179. https://doi.org/10.1007/s00421-015-3245-2
Mohr M, Krustrup P (2013) Heat stress impairs repeated jump ability after competitive elite soccer games. J Strength Cond Res 27(3):683–689. https://doi.org/10.1097/JSC.0b013e31825c3266
Mohr M, Krustrup P, Andersson H, Kirkendal D, Bangsbo J (2008) Match activities of elite women soccer players at different performance levels. J Strength Cond Res 22(2):341–349. https://doi.org/10.1519/JSC.0b013e318165fef6
Mohr M, Krustrup P, Bangsbo J (2003) Match performance of high-standard soccer players with special reference to development of fatigue. J Sports Sci 21(7):519–528. https://doi.org/10.1080/0264041031000071182
Mohr M, Krustrup P, Bangsbo J (2005) Fatigue in soccer: a brief review. J Sports Sci 23(6):593–599. https://doi.org/10.1080/02640410400021286
Mohr M, Mujika I, Santisteban J, Randers MB, Bischoff R, Solano R, Hewitt A, Zubillaga A, Peltola E, Krustrup P (2010) Examination of fatigue development in elite soccer in a hot environment: a multi-experimental approach. Scand J Med Sci Sports 20(Suppl 3):125–132. https://doi.org/10.1111/j.1600-0838.2010.01217.x
Mohr M, Thomassen M, Girard O, Racinais S, Nybo L (2016) Muscle variables of importance for physiological performance in competitive football. Eur J Appl Physiol 116:251. https://doi.org/10.1007/s00421-015-3274-x
Morgans R, Orme P, Anderson L, Drust B, Morton JP (2014) An intensive winter fixture schedule induces a transient fall in salivary IgA in english premier league soccer players. Res Sports Med 22(4):346–354. https://doi.org/10.1080/15438627.2014.944641
Mourot L, Bouhaddi M, Perrey S, Cappelle S, Henriet MT, Wolf JP, Rouillon JD, Regnard J (2004) Decrease in heart rate variability with overtraining: assessment by the Poincaré plot analysis. Clin Physiol Funct Imaging 24(1):10–18. https://doi.org/10.1046/j.1475-0961.2003.00523.x
Mullaney DJ, Kripke DF, Messin S (1980) Wrist-actigraphic estimation of sleep time. Sleep 3(1):83–92. https://doi.org/10.1093/sleep/3.1.83
Myllymäki T, Kyröläinen H, Savolainen K, Hokka L, Jakonen R, Juuti T, Martinmäki K, Kaartinen J, Kinnunen ML, Rusko H (2011) Effects of vigorous late-night exercise on sleep quality and cardiac autonomic activity. J Sleep Res 20(1 Pt 2):146–153. https://doi.org/10.1111/j.1365-2869.2010.00874.x
Myllymäki T, Rusko H, Syväoja H, Juuti T, Kinnunen ML, Kyröläinen H (2012) Effects of exercise intensity and duration on nocturnal heart rate variability and sleep quality. Eur J Appl Physiol 112(3):801–809. https://doi.org/10.1007/s00421-011-2034-9
Nakamura FY, Antunes P, Nunes C, Costa JA, Esco MR, Travassos B (2020) Heart rate variability changes from traditional vs. ultra-short-term recordings in relation to preseason training load and performance in futsal players. J Strength Cond Res 34(10):2974–2981. https://doi.org/10.1519/JSC.0000000000002910
Nédélec M, Dawson B, Dupont G (2019) Influence of night soccer matches on sleep in elite players. J Strength Cond Res 33(1):174–179. https://doi.org/10.1519/JSC.0000000000002906
Nedelec M, Dupont G (2019) The influence of playing position in soccer on the recovery kinetics of cognitive and physical performance. J Sports Med Phys Fitness 59(11):1812–1819. https://doi.org/10.23736/S0022-4707.19.09433-7
Nédélec M, Halson S, Abaidia AE, Ahmaidi S, Dupont G (2015) Stress, sleep and recovery in elite soccer: a critical review of the literature. Sports Med 45(10):1387–1400. https://doi.org/10.1007/s40279-015-0358-z
Nedelec M, McCall A, Carling C, Legall F, Berthoin S, Dupont G (2014) The influence of soccer playing actions on the recovery kinetics after a soccer match. J Strength Cond Res 28(6):1517–1523. https://doi.org/10.1519/JSC.0000000000000293
Nimmo MA, Ekblom B, International Association of Athletics Federations (2007) Fatigue and illness in athletes. J Sports Sci 25(Suppl 1):S93–S102. https://doi.org/10.1080/02640410701607379

Nybo L, Girard O, Mohr M, Knez W, Voss S, Racinais S (2013) Markers of muscle damage and performance recovery after exercise in the heat. Med Sci Sports Exerc 45(5):860–868. https://doi.org/10.1249/MSS.0b013e31827ded04

Ohayon M, Wickwire EM, Hirshkowitz M, Albert SM, Avidan A, Daly FJ, Dauvilliers Y, Ferri R, Fung C, Gozal D, Hazen N, Krystal A, Lichstein K, Mallampalli M, Plazzi G, Rawding R, Scheer FA, Somers V, Vitiello MV (2017) National Sleep Foundation's sleep quality recommendations: first report. Sleep Health 3(1):6–19. https://doi.org/10.1016/j.sleh.2016.11.006

Ohlsson A, Berg L, Ljungberg H, Söderman K, Stålnacke BM (2015) Heart rate distribution during training and a domestic league game in swedish elite female soccer players. Ann Sports Med Res 2(4):1025

Pagani M, Lombardi F, Guzzetti S, Rimoldi O, Furlan R, Pizzinelli P, Sandrone G, Malfatto G, Dell'Orto S, Piccaluga E (1986) Power spectral analysis of heart rate and arterial pressure variabilities as a marker of sympatho-vagal interaction in man and conscious dog. Circ Res 59(2):178–193. https://doi.org/10.1161/01.res.59.2.178

Paquet J, Kawinska A, Carrier J (2007) Wake detection capacity of actigraphy during sleep. Sleep 30(10):1362–1369. https://doi.org/10.1093/sleep/30.10.1362

Parak J, Korhonen I (2013) Accuracy of firstbeat bodyguard 2 beat-to-beat heart rate monitor. White Pap Firstbeat Technol Ltd., Jyväskylä

Parrado E, García MA, Ramos J, Cervantes JC, Rodas G, Capdevila L (2010) Comparison of omega wave system and polar S810i to detect R-R intervals at rest. Int J Sports Med 31(5):336–341. https://doi.org/10.1055/s-0030-1248319

Peterson BT, Chiao P, Pickering E, Freeman J, Zammit GK, Ding Y, Badura LL (2012) Comparison of actigraphy and polysomnography to assess effects of zolpidem in a clinical research unit. Sleep Med 13(4):419–424. https://doi.org/10.1016/j.sleep.2011.12.003

Plews DJ, Laursen PB, Stanley J, Kilding AE, Buchheit M (2013) Training adaptation and heart rate variability in elite endurance athletes: opening the door to effective monitoring. Sports Med 43(9):773–781. https://doi.org/10.1007/s40279-013-0071-8

Postolache TT, Hung TM, Rosenthal RN, Soriano JJ, Montes F, Stiller JW (2005) Sports chronobiology consultation: from the lab to the arena. Clin Sports Med 24(2):415–xiv. https://doi.org/10.1016/j.csm.2005.01.001

Pumprla J, Howorka K, Groves D, Chester M, Nolan J (2002) Functional assessment of heart rate variability: physiological basis and practical applications. Int J Cardiol 84(1):1–14. https://doi.org/10.1016/s0167-5273(02)00057-8

Rae DE, Stephenson KJ, Roden LC (2015) Factors to consider when assessing diurnal variation in sports performance: the influence of chronotype and habitual training time-of-day. Eur J Appl Physiol 115(6):1339–1349. https://doi.org/10.1007/s00421-015-3109-9

Rampinini E, Bosio A, Ferraresi I, Petruolo A, Morelli A, Sassi A (2011) Match-related fatigue in soccer players. Med Sci Sports Exerc 43(11):2161–2170. https://doi.org/10.1249/MSS.0b013e31821e9c5c

Roach GD, Schmidt WF, Aughey RJ, Bourdon PC, Soria R, Claros JC, Garvican-Lewis LA, Buchheit M, Simpson BM, Hammond K, Kley M, Wachsmuth N, Gore CJ, Sargent C (2013) The sleep of elite athletes at sea level and high altitude: a comparison of sea-level natives and high-altitude natives (ISA3600). Br J Sports Med 47(Suppl 1(Suppl 1)):i114–i120. https://doi.org/10.1136/bjsports-2013-092843

Roberts S, Teo WP, Warmington SA (2019) Effects of training and competition on the sleep of elite athletes: a systematic review and meta-analysis. Br J Sports Med 53(8):513–522. https://doi.org/10.1136/bjsports-2018-099322

Robey E, Dawson B, Halson S, Gregson W, Goodman C, Eastwood P (2014) Sleep quantity and quality in elite youth soccer players: a pilot study. Eur J Sport Sci 14(5):410–417. https://doi.org/10.1080/17461391.2013.843024

Rollo I, Impellizzeri FM, Zago M, Iaia FM (2014) Effects of 1 versus 2 games a week on physical and subjective scores of subelite soccer players. Int J Sports Physiol Perform 9(3):425–431. https://doi.org/10.1123/ijspp.2013-0288

Roomkham S, Lovell D, Cheung J, Perrin D (2018) Promises and challenges in the use of consumer-grade devices for sleep monitoring. IEEE Rev Biomed Eng 11:53–67. https://doi.org/10.1109/RBME.2018.2811735

Saltin B (1973) Metabolic fundamentals in exercise. Med Sci Sports 5(3):137–146. https://www.ncbi.nlm.nih.gov/pubmed/4270581

Sargent C, Halson S, Roach GD (2014b) Sleep or swim? Early-morning training severely restricts the amount of sleep obtained by elite swimmers. Eur J Sport Sci 14(Suppl 1):S310–S315. https://doi.org/10.1080/17461391.2012.696711

Sargent C, Lastella M, Halson SL, Roach GD (2014a) The impact of training schedules on the sleep and fatigue of elite athletes. Chronobiol Int 31(10):1160–1168. https://doi.org/10.3109/07420528.2014.957306

Sargent C, Lastella M, Halson SL, Roach GD (2016) The validity of activity monitors for measuring sleep in elite athletes. J Sci Med Sport 19(10):848–853. https://doi.org/10.1016/j.jsams.2015.12.007

Shaffer F, McCraty R, Zerr CL (2014) A healthy heart is not a metronome: an integrative review of the heart's anatomy and heart rate variability. Front Psychol 5:1040. https://doi.org/10.3389/fpsyg.2014.01040

Signal TL, Gale J, Gander PH (2005) Sleep measurement in flight crew: comparing actigraphic and subjective estimates to polysomnography. Aviat Space Environ Med 76(11):1058–1063

Silva JR, Rumpf MC, Hertzog M, Castagna C, Farooq A, Girard O, Hader K (2018) Acute and residual soccer match-related fatigue: a systematic review and meta-analysis. Sports Med 48(3):539–583. https://doi.org/10.1007/s40279-017-0798-8

Stanley J, Peake JM, Buchheit M (2013) Consecutive days of cold water immersion: effects on cycling performance and heart rate variability. Eur J Appl Physiol 113(2):371–384. https://doi.org/10.1007/s00421-012-2445-2

Tarvainen MP, Niskanen JP, Lipponen JA, Ranta-Aho PO, Karjalainen PA (2014) Kubios HRV—heart rate variability analysis software. Comput Methods Prog Biomed 113(1):210–220. https://doi.org/10.1016/j.cmpb.2013.07.024

Taylor SR, Rogers GG, Driver HS (1997) Effects of training volume on sleep, psychological, and selected physiological profiles of elite female swimmers. Med Sci Sports Exerc 29(5):688–693. https://doi.org/10.1097/00005768-199705000-00016

Thorlund JB, Aagaard P, Madsen K (2009) Rapid muscle force capacity changes after soccer match play. Int J Sports Med 30(4):273–278. https://doi.org/10.1055/s-0028-1104587

Thorpe RT, Strudwick AJ, Buchheit M, Atkinson G, Drust B, Gregson W (2015) Monitoring fatigue during the in-season competitive phase in elite soccer players. Int J Sports Physiol Perform 10(8):958–964. https://doi.org/10.1123/ijspp.2015-0004

Tryon WW (2004) Issues of validity in actigraphic sleep assessment. Sleep 27(1):158–165. https://doi.org/10.1093/sleep/27.1.158

Vigh-Larsen JF, Dalgas U, Andersen TB (2018) Position-specific acceleration and deceleration profiles in elite youth and senior soccer players. J Strength Cond Res 32(4):1114–1122. https://doi.org/10.1519/JSC.0000000000001918

Vitale JA, Banfi G, Galbiati A, Ferini-Strambi L, La Torre A (2019) Effect of a night game on Actigraphy-based sleep quality and perceived recovery in top-level volleyball athletes. Int J Sports Physiol Perform 14(2):265–269. https://doi.org/10.1123/ijspp.2018-0194

Wallén MB, Hasson D, Theorell T, Canlon B, Osika W (2012) Possibilities and limitations of the polar RS800 in measuring heart rate variability at rest. Eur J Appl Physiol 112(3):1153–1165. https://doi.org/10.1007/s00421-011-2079-9

Walsh NP, Halson SL, Sargent C, Roach GD, Nédélec M, Gupta L, Leeder J, Fullagar HH, Coutts AJ, Edwards BJ, Pullinger SA, Robertson CM, Burniston JG, Lastella M, Le Meur Y, Hausswirth C, Bender AM, Grandner MA, Samuels CH (2020) Sleep and the athlete: narrative review and 2021 expert consensus recommendations. Br J Sports Med:bjsports-2020-102025. https://doi.org/10.1136/bjsports-2020-102025

Waterhouse J, Atkinson G, Edwards B, Reilly T (2007) The role of a short post-lunch nap in improving cognitive, motor, and sprint performance in participants with partial sleep deprivation. J Sports Sci 25(14):1557–1566. https://doi.org/10.1080/02640410701244983

Watson AM (2017) Sleep and athletic performance. Curr Sports Med Rep 16(6):413–418. https://doi.org/10.1249/JSR.0000000000000418

Watson NF, Badr MS, Belenky G, Bliwise DL, Buxton OM, Buysse D, Dinges DF, Gangwisch J, Grandner MA, Kushida C, Malhotra RK, Martin JL, Patel SR, Quan SF, Tasali E (2015) Recommended amount of sleep for a healthy adult: a joint consensus statement of the American Academy of sleep medicine and Sleep Research Society. Sleep 38(6):843–844. https://doi.org/10.5665/sleep.4716

Weippert M, Kumar M, Kreuzfeld S, Arndt D, Rieger A, Stoll R (2010) Comparison of three mobile devices for measuring R-R intervals and heart rate variability: polar S810i, Suunto t6 and an ambulatory ECG system. Eur J Appl Physiol 109(4):779–786. https://doi.org/10.1007/s00421-010-1415-9

Injury Prevention

6

Kobe C. Houtmeyers and Arne Jaspers

Soccer is a running-based invasion team sport and is characterized by repeated high-intensity efforts and body contacts between players. These characteristics make soccer players vulnerable for injury, which negatively affect health and performance. That is why injury prevention is an important part of the training process in soccer. In this chapter, we discuss the available evidence on injury prevention in soccer and we focus specifically on the relation between training load and injury risk. Load monitoring practices currently receive much attention in the context of injury prevention. However, in this chapter, we critically discuss the current state of evidence that supports these practices. This reflection does not imply that load monitoring is useless but aims to situate it within the bigger picture of injury prevention.

6.1 Injury Epidemiology in Soccer

Soccer is a running-based team sport that involves repeated ball handling actions and (sub) maximal efforts such as accelerations, decelerations, changes in direction, and jumps (Harper et al. 2019). In addition, soccer is an invasion team sport which means that body contact between players is part of the game. These characteristics explain the high injury rate in soccer.

The UEFA Elite Club Injury Study provides an annual report on the injury patterns in European elite soccer (UEFA 2019). In the 2018–2019 season, an average of 43 injuries per team was reported. Of these injuries, 47% occurred during training sessions (1.7 injuries for every 1000 training hours), while 53% occurred during match sessions (21.0 injuries for every 1000 match hours). The most common type

K. C. Houtmeyers · A. Jaspers (✉)
KU Leuven, Faculty of Movement and Rehabilitation Sciences, Leuven, Belgium
e-mail: kobe.houtmeyers@kuleuven.be; arne.jaspers@kuleuven.be

J. M. Oliva Lozano, L. P. Ardigò (eds.), *Training Load in Professional Soccer*,
https://doi.org/10.1007/978-3-031-52087-7_6

of injury were muscle injuries (33%) followed by ligament injuries (21%). The thigh (34%), knee (12%), and hip/groin (11%) were the most affected body zones. The majority of injuries were noncontact injuries (68%) and injury severity was classified as minimal (1–3 days absence, 19%), mild (4–7 days absence, 23%), moderate (8–28 days, 42%), and severe (>28 days, 16%).

The impact of injuries on team performance is also described based on data from the UEFA Injury Study (Hägglund et al. 2013). A lower injury incidence was associated with an increased number of points per domestic league match. A lower injury burden, which combines incidence and severity, was associated with a higher final league ranking and a better performance in European cup competitions. The high injury incidence, the negative impact on performance, and the social responsibility of keeping players healthy explain the importance of injury prevention in soccer.

6.2 Injury Registration in Soccer

The accurate registration of injuries at the club or federation level is an important first step in injury prevention. Guidelines for registering injuries in sport were provided by an expert panel that was commissioned by the International Olympic Committee (Bahr et al. 2020). It is beyond the scope of this book chapter to explain these methods in detail, but we consider some aspects as important to mention.

A first aspect is the injury definition. Injuries can be defined as any medical complaint that reduces the normal state of full health, irrespective of its consequences. However, studies on injury prevention often include only time-loss injuries. These injuries result in the inability to complete current or future training and match sessions. The focus on this injury definition can be explained by the greater impact of these types of injuries on health and performance. However, players often suffer from minor physical complaints that do not result in time-loss but require medical attention. These injuries may impact performance and may predispose players in developing time-loss injuries (Whalan et al. 2020). From the perspective of early detection and prevention, it may therefore be advised to apply a broad injury registration approach, including both time-loss and medical attention injuries. This approach requires a greater time investment which could be minimized by using digital surveillance systems and questionnaires (Clarsen et al. 2020).

A second aspect is the type of variable that is used to describe the impact of injuries on the player, club, or federation. The most common variable is injury incidence, which reflects the rate of injury occurrence. This variable can be used to monitor trends in injury occurrence or can provide insight into the most common types of injuries in a particular sport such as soccer. However, injury incidence does not provide information about the severity of the injuries. Severity can be described using different variables such as the number of days that the players suffer from injury, whether or not leading to time-loss, or the economic costs (e.g., salary) resulting from injury. In more severe cases, variables such as performance recovery and sports retirement rate are also useful to monitor. Including information about injury severity is important to make informed decisions about injury prevention

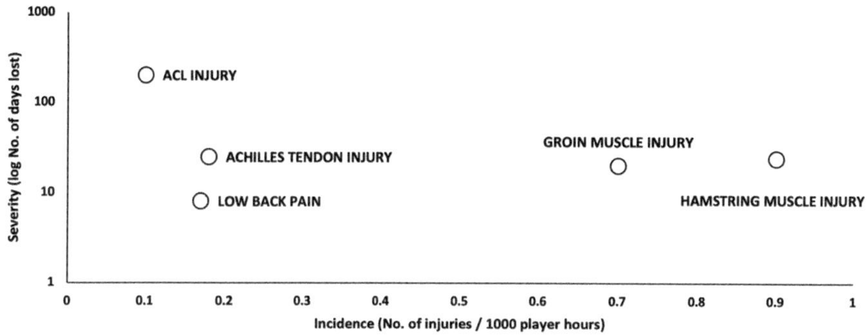

Fig. 6.1 Risk matrix showing the combined impact of incidence and severity (i.e., injury burden). (Based on data from the UEFA Elite Club Injury Study and adapted from Bahr et al. (2018))

(Bahr et al. 2018). This variable can, for example, be used to prioritize injury prevention practices. If two types of injuries occur at a similar rate, it may be obvious to prioritize practices related to preventing the type of injury with the highest severity. Such information can be visualized in a risk matrix (Fig. 6.1).

Take-Home Messages

- Injury registration is a first step towards injury prevention. In addition to time-loss injuries, it is also advised to monitor less severe complaints.
- Digital surveillance systems and questionnaires may aid in efficiently registering injury data.
- Injury patterns can be visualized in a risk matrix that combines injury incidence and severity. The matrix can be used to prioritize injury prevention practices.

6.3 Injury Causation

The next step in injury prevention is the identification of the mechanisms that cause injury. The current scientific frameworks highlight the importance of load in injury causation (Windt and Gabbett 2017). However, the relation between training load and injury risk is influenced by other risk factors, which can be either internal or external to the player (Windt et al. 2017). Internal variables reflect the individual characteristics of the player and can be divided into modifiable (e.g., strength) and non-modifiable variables (e.g., anatomy). The same high-speed running load may, for example, be better tolerated by a player with high eccentric hamstring strength compared to a player with reduced strength (Buckthorpe et al. 2019). During training or match sessions, players are exposed to external variables which can be of human (e.g., tackles) or environmental origin (e.g., surface). The relation between high-speed running load and hamstring injury risk may, for example, be different when playing on natural grass compared to artificial grass (Buckthorpe et al. 2019).

In 2017, a publication of Vanrenterghem and colleagues highlighted the importance of the biomechanical load in injury causation (Vanrenterghem et al. 2017). According to the authors, the biomechanical load is often overlooked in load monitoring. This can be explained by the difficulty of measuring biomechanical loads during training and match sessions (Verheul et al. 2020). To improve biomechanical load monitoring, Kalkhoven et al. (2020) developed a detailed framework for stress-related, strain-related, and overuse athletic injury. The main idea behind this framework is that the immediate or repetitive application of biomechanical load results in tissue damage. When the capacity of the tissue to withstand this damage is exceeded, tissue failure can occur resulting in an injury. The applied load can be divided into stress and strain. Stress refers to the internal forces experienced by the tissue. Strain is defined as the amount of deformation or length change in the tissue in the direction of an applied force. It is still not possible to quantify stress and strain during field-based training sessions (Verheul et al. 2020). External load variables such as the distance covered or the number of sprints completed are often used as a derivative to estimate the biomechanical load. Other variables such as Player Load™ are also proposed as more specific measures of the biomechanical load (Barreira et al. 2017). However, it is important to keep in mind that the same external load can result in a different biomechanical internal load (i.e., stress and strain). For example, the same running velocity for two players may impact the players differently on the musculoskeletal system because of differences in the individual physiology (e.g., muscle mass) and the corresponding tissue-specific mechanical properties (e.g., tissue lengths). Therefore, caution is warranted when interpreting these external load variables in relation to injury risk.

Take-Home Messages

- Different theoretical frameworks are proposed about injury causation in sport. All these frameworks emphasize the interplay between the individual characteristics of the player and the training load. This indicates the importance of both screening and load management.
- Noncontact injuries are caused by immediate or repetitive excessive biomechanical stresses and strain. Future research and practice has to focus on developing tools to monitor these biomechanical loads.

6.4 The Association Between Training Load and Injury Risk

Research on injury prevention in soccer mainly focuses on the association between training load and injury risk. It is important to emphasize that this type of analysis does not provide strong evidence for causation. A short example to illustrate this distinction: it can be that the risk of food poisoning is associated with having a lower age, but this does not mean that having a lower age causes food poisoning. The identification of clear causal relations is complex and often difficult to address in an applied setting in which it is not possible to design a study with high experimental control (Stovitz et al. 2019). Therefore, the current research on load and injury risk must be evaluated on the level of association. To examine associations between load and injury risk, load variables (e.g., distance covered, rating of perceived exertion, heart rate) are often modelled as cumulative load, relative load, and load variation.

6.4.1 Cumulative Load

It is the averaged or summated load over a given time window and is generally expressed per day, week, month, or periodization cycle. To monitor the cumulative load from day to day, rolling averages (or sums) are used. However, these methods have two limitations (Menaspà 2017). First, averages do not consider the variation in load during a given period. Second, rolling averages do not consider the decline of the effect of load over time. To address this issue, it may be appropriate to give a higher weighting to more recent loads. The use of exponentially weighted moving averages (EWMA) was therefore proposed and can, for example, be calculated as follows (Williams et al. 2017):

$$\mathrm{EWMA}_{\mathrm{today}} = \mathrm{Load}_{\mathrm{today}}\ \mathrm{X}\,\lambda_{\mathrm{a}} + \left(\left(1-\lambda_{\mathrm{a}}\right)\mathrm{X}\,\mathrm{EWMA}_{\mathrm{yesterday}}\right)$$

$$\mathrm{met}\,\lambda_{\mathrm{a}} = 2/\left(\mathrm{N}+1\right)$$

with N = chosen time decay constant.

We notice that the calculation of EWMA is just an analytic approach and does not reflect any physical recovery mechanism as is sometimes thought.

Intuitively, one can reason that injury risk increases with higher cumulative loads because players exceed their load tolerance in such scenarios. In extreme cases, this association may indeed be present. However, such scenarios are rare in soccer. In general, the available evidence shows no strong and consistent association between cumulative load and injury risk (Jaspers et al. 2017). Although there is no strong evidence, we still advise to use load thresholds, specific to the sport (level), to compare the maximally planned training load with the actual training load (Impellizzeri et al. 2020a, b). These thresholds are ideally individualized for every player and context because other variables such as injury history may impact players' load tolerance. If planned appropriately, high cumulative loads increase players' fitness and load tolerance. Therefore, it is advised to continuously adapt thresholds by estimating players' load tolerance. In this context, the application of relative load variables holds promise because these variables reflect the balance between cumulative load and load tolerance.

6.4.2 Relative Load

The most discussed relative load variable of the 2000s is the acute/chronic workload ratio (ACWR; Gabbett 2016). This variable was originally proposed as the ratio between the cumulative load averaged over the last 7 days (acute load; load) and the cumulative load averaged over the last 28 days (chronic load; load tolerance). An ACWR value higher than 1.0 is interpreted as "the player is training harder than he is normally used to," and vice versa. The association between ACWR and injury risk was described as a U-shaped curve, with an increased injury risk below values of 0.8 and above 1.3. Given its simplicity and plausibility, the ACWR became a popular variable in sports science, something that is currently under debate. Questions were raised about the validity of the variable because there is no high-level evidence relating ACWR to injury risk (Wang et al. 2020). In addition, the ACWR was criticized for its statistical correctness (Lolli et al. 2019). It is beyond the scope of this book chapter to explain this debate in more detail. For more information, we refer to Gabbett (2020) and Impellizzeri et al. (2020a, b).

Taken together, the idea of relative load variables seems plausible because it may reflect the balance between load and load tolerance in a single value. From a scientific point of view, we advise to be careful when interpreting variables such as the ACWR. Similar to cumulative load variables, we advise to apply a multifactorial approach when interpreting relative load variables, with load management being informed by general training principles that can be adapted to every player and context (Impellizzeri et al. 2020a, b).

6.4.3 Load Variation

Relative load variables are useful for monitoring the progression in load because one can expect that a rapid progression in load increases injury risk. Although this could seem to advise against load variation, insufficient variation (i.e., high monotony) may also be a risk factor for injury. The concept of load monotony was introduced in injury risk research by Foster (1998), inspired by a study on racehorses (Bruin et al. 1994). In this study, racehorses were exposed to a hard day–easy day training cycle. It was shown that racehorses developed more overtraining symptoms if the load was increased on the easy day (i.e., higher monotony) compared to an increased load on the hard day (i.e., lower monotony). Recently, some studies were published that examined the association between load variation and injury risk in elite soccer. Brink et al. (2010) demonstrated that a higher weekly monotony was related to an increased risk of traumatic injury. However, Delecroix et al. (2019) showed that injury risk was decreased when 4-weekly monotony was increased. These contrasting results could be explained by the injury definition, the time window over which monotony was calculated, or the type of population (youth versus senior players). Therefore, similar to cumulative and relative load variables, we conclude that the concept of load variation is conceptually plausible but high-level evidence about its relationship with injury risk is not available.

6.4.4 Reasons for Lacking Evidence

There are several explanations for the lack of strong and consistent associations between load variables and injury risk. The main explanation is that injury causation is multifactorial and complex (Bittencourt et al. 2016). This means that multiple variables interact with each other in a dynamic way. Isolated load models such as cumulative loads, ACWR, and monotony scores fail to recognize this complexity. Therefore, we advise to combine information from different variables to inform decisions on injury prevention. However, when the complexity of data increases, the generated information can exceed the capacity of the human brain to accurately process this information. Artificial intelligence methods such as machine learning could therefore be helpful to better unravel patterns in complex data (Rommers et al. 2020; Rossi et al. 2018). A second explanation is that the amount of data that is collected in soccer is rather small to identify strong associations. Most studies rely on monitoring observations from a single soccer club over one or multiple seasons. Therefore, these studies include a limited number of injuries and are therefore often not able to examine associations between load and specific injury types. Studies including observations from multiple clubs over multiple seasons are therefore needed. A final explanation is the lack of internal biomechanical load data. Typical load variables such as high-speed running distance only provide indirect insight into the biomechanical mechanisms that are associated with injury risk such as muscular strain and stress (Verheul et al. 2020). Future research should validate methods to measure these mechanisms during field-based training sessions.

Take-Home Messages

- Training load can be modelled as cumulative load, relative load, and load variation. All these variables provide information about the trend in load over a given period and are ideally interpreted using general training principles.
- There are no strong and consistent associations between single training load variables and injury risk. A multifactorial approach is advised to embrace the complexity of injury causation.
- Individualization is key in injury prevention. Load management is ideally based on an individualized injury risk profile.
- Artificial intelligence methods may provide more insight in the complex nature of injury causation in the near future.

6.5 It Is Not All About Load

In the absence of strong evidence, it is useful to use the opinion of experienced practitioners to design injury prevention practices. In 2020, a Delphi study was conducted to gather opinions and to assess agreement between experienced sports practitioners of elite European soccer clubs (McCall et al. 2020). The management of high-speed and sprint load was considered very effective in preventing muscle injuries, with 72% consensus between practitioners. This confirms the perceived importance of managing training load, especially with regard to high-speed activity which induces a higher muscular strain and stress. Exercises with an eccentric focus were considered to be effective with 100% consensus. These exercises may be preferred because reduced eccentric strength and short fascicle lengths can increase injury risk. Exercises with a concentric and isometric focus were considered as somewhat effective, similar to other exercises such as dynamic and static flexibility, core stability, and plyometric exercises. All these exercise ratings had more than 75% consensus. Although these findings are only supported by weak evidence, it does provide insight into what is perceived as best practice.

It is clear that injury prevention programs must be tailored to the specific needs of the player. Periodic health examinations are therefore common practice in elite soccer to generate an individual injury risk profile (McCall et al. 2016). Because there is no evidence supporting the use of isolated test results to accurately determine injury risk, a broad range of medical, musculoskeletal, and performance tests are often applied (Hughes et al. 2017). Based on these tests, players can be categorized into low, medium, and high risk for a given type of injury, with cutoff thresholds being determined based on experience, between-player, and within-player comparisons. We advise to not consider these periodic health examinations as baseline measurements in which all players are asymptomatic and injury-free. Players have their own injury history which continues to be present as most musculoskeletal problems are transient and chronic (Hughes et al. 2018). It is therefore useful to analyze test results in consideration of players' injury history and current medical condition. This indicates that it may be better to analyze trends instead of single values.

Take-Home Messages

- The management of high-speed training load and the use of eccentric strength exercises is perceived by experienced practitioners as an effective muscle injury prevention practice in soccer.
- Periodic health examinations may provide insight to individualize injury prevention practices in soccer.

6.6 Summary

Recent studies such as the UEFA Elite Club Injury Study have provided insight into the injury patterns in soccer. This information can be used to prioritize injury prevention practices and can be used to evaluate the effectiveness of these practices by monitoring injury rates. The current theoretical frameworks have a pronounced focus on the association between load and injury risk. However, we outlined that there is no strong evidence of this association in soccer. This can be explained by the complexity of injury causation and the current lack of methods to collect more precise data about the internal biomechanical load. Therefore, we advise to be careful in interpreting isolated load variables. A multifactorial approach, consisting of both screening and load data, is recommended to determine injury risk. Data can support decisions on injury prevention but have to be interpreted based on general training principles.

References

Bahr R, Clarsen B, Ekstrand J (2018) Why we should focus on the burden of injuries and illnesses, not just their incidence. Br J Sports Med 52(16):1018–1021. https://doi.org/10.1136/bjsports-2017-098160

Bahr R, Clarsen B, Derman W, Dvorak J, Emery CA, Finch CF, Hägglund M, Junge A, Kemp S, Khan KM, Marshall SW, Meeuwisse W, Mountjoy M, Orchard JW, Pluim B, Quarrie KL, Reider B, Schwellnus M, Soligard T, Stokes KA, Chamari K (2020) International olympic committee consensus statement: methods for recording and reporting of epidemiological data on injury and illness in sport 2020 (including STROBE extension for sport injury and illness surveillance (STROBE-SIIS)). Br J Sports Med 54(7):372–389. https://doi.org/10.1136/bjsports-2019-101969

Barreira P, Robinson MA, Drust B, Nedergaard N, Raja Azidin R, Vanrenterghem J (2017) Mechanical player load™ using trunk-mounted accelerometry in football: is it a reliable, task- and player-specific observation? J Sports Sci 35(17):1674–1681. https://doi.org/10.1080/02640414.2016.122901

Bittencourt N, Meeuwisse WH, Mendonça LD, Nettel-Aguirre A, Ocarino JM, Fonseca ST (2016) Complex systems approach for sports injuries: moving from risk factor identification to injury pattern recognition-narrative review and new concept. Br J Sports Med 50(21):1309–1314. https://doi.org/10.1136/bjsports-2015-095850

Brink MS, Visscher C, Arends S, Zwerver J, Post WJ, Lemmink KA (2010) Monitoring stress and recovery: new insights for the prevention of injuries and illnesses in elite youth soccer players. Br J Sports Med 44(11):809–815. https://doi.org/10.1136/bjsm.2009.069476

Bruin G, Kuipers H, Keizer HA, Vander Vusse GJ (1994) Adaptation and overtraining in horses subjected to increasing training loads. J Appl Physiol (1985) 76(5):1908–1913. https://doi.org/10.1152/jappl.1994.76.5.1908

Buckthorpe M, Wright S, Bruce-Low S, Nanni G, Sturdy T, Gross AS, Bowen L, Styles B, Della Villa S, Davison M, Gimpel M (2019) Recommendations for hamstring injury prevention in elite football: translating research into practice. Br J Sports Med 53(7):449–456. https://doi.org/10.1136/bjsports-2018-099616

Clarsen B, Bahr R, Myklebust G, Andersson SH, Docking SI, Drew M, Finch CF, Fortington LV, Harøy J, Khan KM, Moreau B, Moore IS, Møller M, Nabhan D, Nielsen RO, Pasanen K, Schwellnus M, Soligard T, Verhagen E (2020) Improved reporting of overuse injuries and health problems in sport: an update of the Oslo sport trauma research center questionnaires. Br J Sports Med 54(7):390–396. https://doi.org/10.1136/bjsports-2019-101337

Delecroix B, Mccall A, Dawson B, Berthoin S, Dupont G (2019) Workload monotony, strain and non-contact injury incidence in professional football players. Sci Med Footb 3(2):105–108. https://doi.org/10.1080/24733938.2018.1508881

Foster C (1998) Monitoring training in athletes with reference to overtraining syndrome. Med Sci Sports Exerc 30(7):1164–1168. https://doi.org/10.1097/00005768-199807000-00023

Gabbett TJ (2016) The training-injury prevention paradox: should athletes be training smarter and harder? Br J Sports Med 50(5):273–280. https://doi.org/10.1136/bjsports-2015-09578

Gabbett TJ (2020) The training-performance puzzle: how can the past inform future training directions? J Athl Train 55(9):874–884. https://doi.org/10.4085/1062/6050.422.1

Hägglund M, Waldén M, Magnusson H, Kristenson K, Bengtsson H, Ekstrand J (2013) Injuries affect team performance negatively in professional football: an 11-year follow-up of the UEFA champions league injury study. Br J Sports Med 47(12):738–742. https://doi.org/10.1136/bjsports-2013-092215

Harper DJ, Carling C, Kiely J (2019) High-intensity acceleration and deceleration demands in elite team sports competitive match play: a systematic review and meta-analysis of observational studies. Sports Med 49(12):1923–1947. https://doi.org/10.1007/s40279-019-01170-1

Hughes T, Sergeant JC, Parkes MJ, Callaghan MJ (2017) Prognostic factors for specific lower extremity and spinal musculoskeletal injuries identified through medical screening and training load monitoring in professional football (soccer): a systematic review. BMJ Open Sport Exerc Med 3(1):e000263. https://doi.org/10.1136/bmjsem-2017-00026

Hughes T, Sergeant JC, van der Windt DA, Riley R, Callaghan MJ (2018) Periodic health examination and injury prediction in professional football (soccer): theoretically, the prognosis is good. Sports Med 48(11):2443–2448. https://doi.org/10.1007/s40279-018-0928-y

Impellizzeri FM, McCall A, Ward P, Bornn L, Coutts AJ (2020a) Training load and its role in injury prevention, part 2: conceptual and methodologic pitfalls. J Athl Train 55(9):893–901. https://doi.org/10.4085/1062-6050-501-19

Impellizzeri FM, Menaspà P, Coutts AJ, Kalkhoven J, Menaspà MJ (2020b) Training load and its role in injury prevention, part I: back to the future. J Athl Train 55(9):885–892. https://doi.org/10.4085/1062-6050-500-19

Jaspers A, Brink MS, Probst SG, Frencken WG, Helsen WF (2017) Relationships between training load indicators and training outcomes in professional soccer. Sports Med 47(3):533–544. https://doi.org/10.1007/s40279-016-0591-0

Kalkhoven JT, Watsford ML, Impellizzeri FM (2020) A conceptual model and detailed framework for stress-related, strain-related, and overuse athletic injury. J Sci Med Sport 23(8):726–734. https://doi.org/10.1016/j.jsams.2020.02.002

Lolli L, Batterham AM, Hawkins R, Kelly DM, Strudwick AJ, Thorpe RT, Gregson W, Atkinson G (2019) The acute-to-chronic workload ratio: an inaccurate scaling index for an unnecessary normalisation process? Br J Sports Med 53(24):1510–1512. https://doi.org/10.1136/bjsports-2017-09888

McCall A, Dupont G, Ekstrand J (2016) Injury prevention strategies, coach compliance and player adherence of 33 of the UEFA elite club injury study teams: a survey of teams' head medical officers. Br J Sports Med 50(12):725–730. https://doi.org/10.1136/bjsports-2015-095259

McCall A, Pruna R, Van der Horst N, Dupont G, Buchheit M, Coutts AJ, Impellizzeri FM, Fanchini M, EFP-Group (2020) Exercise-based strategies to prevent muscle injury in male elite footballers: an expert-led Delphi survey of 21 practitioners belonging to 18 teams from the big-5 European Leagues. Sports Med 50(9):1667–1681. https://doi.org/10.1007/s40279-020-01315-7

Menaspà P (2017) Are rolling averages a good way to assess training load for injury prevention? Br J Sports Med 51(7):618–619. https://doi.org/10.1136/bjsports-2016-096131

Rommers N, Rössler R, Verhagen E, Vandecasteele F, Verstockt S, Vaeyens R, Lenoir M, D'Hondt E, Witvrouw E (2020) A machine learning approach to assess injury risk in elite youth football players. Med Sci Sports Exerc 52(8):1745–1751. https://doi.org/10.1249/MSS.0000000000002305

Rossi A, Pappalardo L, Cintia P, Iaia FM, Fernàndez J, Medina D (2018) Effective injury forecasting in soccer with GPS training data and machine learning. PLoS One 13(7):e0201264. https://doi.org/10.1371/journal.pone.0201264

Stovitz SD, Verhagen E, Shrier I (2019) Distinguishing between causal and non-causal associations: implications for sports medicine clinicians. Br J Sports Med 53(7):398–399. https://doi.org/10.1136/bjsports-2017-098520

UEFA (2019) UEFA elite club injury study: 2018–2019 season report: team X; https://www.uefa.com/MultimediaFiles/Download/uefaorg/Medical/02/61/67/86/2616786_DOWNLOAD.pdf

Vanrenterghem J, Nedergaard NJ, Robinson MA, Drust B (2017) Training load monitoring in team sports: a novel framework separating physiological and biomechanical load-adaptation pathways. Sports Med 47(11):2135–2142. https://doi.org/10.1007/s40279-017-0714-2

Verheul J, Nedergaard NJ, Vanrenterghem J, Robinson MA (2020) Measuring biomechanical loads in team sports–from lab to field. Sci Med Footb 4(3):246–252. https://doi.org/10.1080/24733938.2019.1709654

Wang C, Vargas JT, Stokes T, Steele R, Shrier I (2020) Analyzing activity and injury: lessons learned from the acute: chronic workload ratio. Sports Med 50(7):1243–1254. https://doi.org/10.1007/s40279-020-01280-1

Whalan M, Lovell R, Sampson JA (2020) Do niggles matter?-increased injury risk following physical complaints in football (soccer). Sci Med Footb 4(3):216–224. https://doi.org/10.1080/24733938.2019.1705996

Williams S, West S, Cross MJ, Stokes KA (2017) Better way to determine the acute:chronic workload ratio? Br J Sports Med 51(3):209–210. https://doi.org/10.1136/bjsports-2016-09658

Windt J, Gabbett TJ (2017) How do training and competition workloads relate to injury? The workload-injury aetiology model. Br J Sports Med 51(5):428–435. https://doi.org/10.1136/bjsports-2016-096040

Windt J, Zumbo BD, Sporer B, MacDonald K, Gabbett TJ (2017) Why do workload spikes cause injuries, and which athletes are at higher risk? Mediators and moderators in workload-injury investigations. Br J Sports Med 51(13):993–994. https://doi.org/10.1136/bjsports-2016-097255

Return to Play

7

Andrea Riboli

The return-to-play decision-making involves multiple stakeholders, including the individual player, the sports medicine team, the coaching staff, and the technical/performance teams. A combination of clinical, functional, and psychological criteria may help to assess the return to preinjury levels. In the early phases of rehabilitation, physio care and gym-based physical preparation are essential to reduce the differences between injured and uninjured body parts. Monitoring the strength development and pain perceptions plays a key role to guide the training prescriptions. In the last phases of rehabilitation, the use of global positioning tracking systems during on-field practice was considered an important tool to progress training load up to the maximal match demands. The workload progression should move from high control to very high unpredictable soccer-specific exercises with an emphasis on high-intensity workload; the training load should achieve the peak performance demands occurring during official matches. Players have to be adapted to the usual training workload typically sustained during the preinjury periods, including volume and intensity occurring during the official match. Additionally, the stakeholders should detect the acute and chronic training-induced physical and psychological adaptations across the whole training routine. These may help to support the decision-making process for a full training participation without restrictions.

7.1 Injury Incidence in Soccer

Soccer is one of the most important sport in the world. Over the years, a lot of research projects have been provided about performance development using strength and conditioning training prescriptions. However, at professional level, also the

A. Riboli (✉)
MilanLab Research Department, AC Milan S.p.A., Milan, Italy
e-mail: riboliandrea@outlook.com

J. M. Oliva Lozano, L. P. Ardigò (eds.), *Training Load in Professional Soccer*,
https://doi.org/10.1007/978-3-031-52087-7_7

injury risk should be considered as a crucial factor affecting the players' performance (Eirale et al. 2017). Soccer involves relatively high risks and rates of injury in both professional adult (Hawkins and Fuller 1999; Hawkins et al. 2001) and youth (Le Gall et al. 2006; Price et al. 2004) players. Nowadays, athletes are playing the game faster and more aggressively than in the past (Andersen et al. 2004), requiring elevated physical fitness levels and more intensive training (Andersen et al. 2004). This might lead to an increase in injury risk during both training and match (Ekstrand et al. 2016). For example, a ~ 4% increment in muscle injuries through a 13-year longitudinal analysis (i.e., from 2001 to 2014) of the UEFA elite football was found (Ekstrand et al. 2016). An 11-year follow-up study of the UEFA Champions League reported that teams with lower injury incidence and greater consistent player's availability performed better reaching a higher rank position during competitions (Hägglund et al. 2013). Similar positive effects of injury reduction were found in Qatari professional football (Eirale et al. 2013).

The most common injury types are strains, sprains, and contusions. The thigh and hamstring are the most frequently injured parts (Pfirrmann et al. 2016). Other common injury locations are the groin, knee, and ankle (Morgan and Oberlander 2001; Waldén et al. 2005). Fractures represent only a small percentage of all injuries (Pfirrmann et al. 2016; Waldén et al. 2005). Within injuries, muscle injuries are reported as one of the major problems facing football players and it is reported to present ~20% of all time-loss injuries at professional level (Ekstrand et al. 2011a).

The total injury incidence in professional soccer players ranged from 2.48 injuries (Ekstrand et al. 2011a) to 9.4 injuries (Waldén et al. 2005) per 1000 h of exposure. The injury rate during competition ranged from 8.7 injuries (Ekstrand et al. 2011a) to 65.9 injuries (Eirale et al. 2012) per 1000 h of exposure, whereas the injury incidence during training ranged from 1.37 injuries (Ekstrand et al. 2011a) to 5.8 injuries (Waldén et al. 2005) per 1000 h of exposure. Therefore, the high injury risks were during match than training (Pfirrmann et al. 2016). Interestingly, a higher injury risk in Asian than European national team level was found (Eirale et al. 2012; Yoon et al. 2004). It was argued that a lower training status puts the players at a higher risk of injury (Gabbett 2016; Yoon et al. 2004). Similarly, it was previously reported that a higher individual fitness status (i.e., high aerobic, anaerobic, and strength levels) may protect against injuries (Gabbett 2016; Lauersen et al. 2018). Additionally, it could be argued that a higher match than training demands might lead to a higher injury incidence. A higher match vs. training demands have been previously reported in English Premier League (Akenhead et al. 2016), French Ligue 1 (Lacome et al. 2018), Reserve Spanish La Liga (Martín-García et al. 2018), Dutch Eredivisie (Stevens et al. 2017), and first Division Portuguese (Castillo et al. 2021) league. However, no current evidences about the link between match vs. training demands and injury occurrence are available. Only a harmful association of sprinting with muscle injury occurrence during official match demands was reported (Gregson et al. 2020). However, practitioners should be aware about these results for injury prevention purposes.

The injury risk and the time-loss at professional level have also a great economic impact (Orchard 2009). The average cost of a first-team top player being injured for

1 month was calculated to be around €500,000 (Ekstrand 2013). In major European football, it was previously reported that an injury could last about ~14 to ~18 days of absence leading to investment losses of about €250,000 to €300,000 for each injured player. In a 16-year follow-up UEFA study, about 22,942 injuries were registered during 494 team seasons reporting that most of these injuries were either mild (i.e., leading to a median absence of 7 days or less, 6440 cases = 42%) or moderate (i.e., median absence: 7–28 days, 56% = 8518 cases) while only few (i.e., 2% = 311 cases) were severe (i.e., median absence of >28 days).

In general, a football team with 25 players can expect about 15 muscle injuries per season. Moreover, in European Clubs competing in UEFA competitions, a 15.3% of reinjury incidence (i.e., 101 of 658) were reported (Waldén et al. 2005). Additionally, reinjuries required more rest than new injuries (Ekstrand et al. 2011b). Therefore, within professional training, a crucial importance is play by a well-designed return-to-play (RTPlay) process that should decrease the time-loss preparing the players to full-time training participation and coach selection for competition. Moreover, RTPlay should play a key role to avoid reinjuries.

7.2 Return to Play in Soccer

Depending on the injury type and severity, athletes' training is either stopped or reduced, resulting in a period of reduced load and resultant detraining. As the athlete progresses through the various rehabilitation phases, training distribution, intensity, and volume should be manipulated to return the athlete in a condition that meets the demands of the competition (Ritchie et al. 2017). A balance between a fast and a good RTPlay is a crucial factor affecting the rehabilitation process (Taberner et al. 2019). A return to full training participation without restrictions but with a "tolerable risk" could lead to a higher reinjury risk than a full training participation with a certain complete scar maturation. The full comprehension of biological maturation should guide training prescriptions and the return to full training participation. However, a certain comprehension of the maturation process is challenging. Therefore, physiological, locomotor, and perceived loads play a key role in training load management and decision-making across the rehabilitation process.

Early reintegration to training and match play following injury increases the risk of reinjury (Taberner et al. 2019). However, having key players available as soon as possible benefits the team (Ekstrand 2013; Hägglund et al. 2013). This is one of the most important factors that may affect the RTPlay decision process in professional football. The RTPlay decision-making process involves multiple stakeholders, including the individual player, the sports medicine team, the coaching staff, and the technical/performance teams. In English Premier League football (Dunlop et al. 2020), ~80% of the clubs adopted a shared decision-making process with at least two people involved at any phase.

Different interests (e.g., economical, performance, medical, etc.) may affect the RTPlay process leading to a highly pressured decision process. All aspects must be combined effectively to facilitate a successful RTPlay (Bisciotti et al. 2019).

The term RTPlay was defined by the American Academy of Orthopaedic Surgeons and the American College of Sports Medicine (Herring et al. 2012, 2013) as:

"The decision-making process of returning an injured or ill athlete to practice or competition. This ultimately leads to medical clearance of an athlete for full participation in sports."

Two consensus statements (Ardern et al. 2016; Bisciotti et al. 2019) stated that the rehabilitation process should be divided into two different concepts of return to training (RTTrain) and RPplay. The RTTrain include each activity for "return to sport practice/training with possible restrictions" and RTPlay means "return to training and competition without restriction." Recently, a worldwide survey of 131 Premier League football teams (Dunlop et al. 2020) defined four different steps for the RTPlay continuum process:

1. Return to high-speed running (RTRun): the period between injury occurring and the player being cleared to run on-field and progresses to high-speed running.
2. Return to train (RTTrain): when the player is allowed to return to on-field unrestricted training.
3. Return to play (RTPlay): when the player is cleared to return to competitive match play with the team (whether selected or not).
4. Return-to-performance (RTPerf): when the player returned to preinjury levels of performance (or higher).

The worldwide surveys highlighted that a continuum approach to guide RTPlay using a combination of clinical, functional, and psychological criteria was most common at RTRun and RTTrain, while functional criteria were consistently assessed across all phases. Across the later phases of the RTPlay, greater focus was placed on the assessment of psychological readiness (Dunlop et al. 2020).

It was also suggested (Bisciotti et al. 2019) that the RTTrain and RTPlay process must be supported by:

1. Identification of appropriate clinical tests dependent on the type of injury.
2. Identification of appropriate imaging protocols dependent on the type of injuries.
3. Identification of appropriate laboratory tests specific to the functional deficit for the type of injury.
4. Identification of appropriate field tests specific to the functional deficit for the type of injury.

The test battery should consider physical, physiological, neuromuscular, and functional individual assessment and depends on the time-loss and the recurrent time-loss injury (Bisciotti et al. 2019; Dunlop et al. 2020). Also, the "tolerable risk" (Bisciotti et al. 2019) or "the strategic assessment of risk and risk tolerance" (Ardern et al. 2016) is reported as a crucial issue defined as the maximum level of acceptable risk during a short or long RTTrain process. The tolerable or strategic assessment of the risks is an equally divided decision taken by the medical staff, performance staff, technical staff, team management, and player. This risk should be calculated on objective measures such as clinical examination, imaging, functional tests, etc.

The functional tests should be both general and sport-specific and should assess:

1. The force required during muscle contraction.
2. The speed required during movements.
3. The power expressed during movement.
4. The type of movement required.
5. The specificity to sport-specific requirement and to the movement that previously caused the injury (e.g., high-speed running, sprint, change of direction, kicking, etc.).

For the RTTrain and RTPlay process, subjective criteria to determine the individual mood of each player may also be considered. For example, pain values daily reported using the visual analogue scale and/or wellness scales are acceptable. The presence of pain could highlight an incomplete healing suggesting cautions in training prescriptions during the RTTrain/RTPlay process (Ardern et al. 2016; Zambaldi et al. 2017).

Similarly, the RTPlay process should be based on objective assessment to determine if the athletes are fit enough to play without any reinjury risks and to return to full training and competitions without any restrictions. A worldwide experts' panel (van der Horst et al. 2017) defined the following criteria to support RTPlay decision:

1. Medical staff clearance.
2. Similar mobility and flexibility of the injured side compared with preinjury data and/or uninjured side, depending on which data are available or the most reliable for the individual player according to the performance and medical staff.
3. Performance (i.e., flexibility, strength, and functional assessment) on field tests compared with the preinjury individual data (>90% than preinjury data) or with minimum required standards for the team and/or specific population.
4. 0–10% difference between the injured and uninjured side.
5. Psychological readiness (i.e., mental attitude).
6. Absence of pain.

Other experts' consensus (Zambaldi et al. 2017) also defined other criteria to support RTPlay decision, as follows:

1. Perform maximal sprints achieving maximal linear speed (i.e., 100% consensus).
2. Complete at least one football-specific field testing session at maximal performance and under fatigue conditions (i.e., 100% consensus).
3. Perform a progressive running plan with running performance matching preinjury level (i.e., 100% consensus).
4. No pain in the muscle (i.e., ~94% consensus).
5. Player's self-reported feeling of confidence and readiness to RTPlay (i.e., ~94% consensus).
6. Full muscle strength, equal to the uninjured side and/or to preinjury benchmark values (i.e., ~94% consensus).

With regard to performance field testing, different experts' panels defined as eligible different assessments. Repeated sprint ability test, single-leg bridge, and acceleration drills reached >70% consensus and were reported as the eligible assessment for RTPlay by van der Horst et al. (2017), while, ~68% to ~33% of the consensus was achieved for T-test, 40-m sprint, H-test, 20-m sprint, Nordic hamstring exercise, triple hop test, muscular endurance, yo-yo/shuttle test, speed testing, functional movement screen, and single hop test. Overall, a clear consensus was achieved about the use of objective data to assess individual readiness for RTPlay; conversely, no similar consensus was reached about the more reliable testing procedures. The great consensus (i.e., 82%) to test players' readiness was achieved by the use of rehabilitation protocols targeted on position-specific match demands (i.e., determined by global positioning system [GPS] technologies; van der Horst et al. 2017). Other experts' panels showed the greater consensus (i.e., ~100%) to perform maximal sprint assessment using GPS technology based on the player's self-reported maximal perceived effort on 10- and 30-m timed acceleration tests (Zambaldi et al. 2017). Bisciotti et al. (2019) stated that functional tests must attempt to simulate real-time game situations that replicate force, speed, and power within position-specific movement with a particular emphasis on the movement that caused injury. Performance on field testing was considered vital by another expert panel (van der Horst et al. 2017) when assessing RTPlay readiness, as it mimics the actual sports requirements. Additionally, to perform at least one football-specific testing session at maximal performance under fatigue conditions achieved a good experts' agreement (Ardern et al. 2016; Bisciotti et al. 2019; van der Horst et al. 2017; Zambaldi et al. 2017). During the last part of the RTPlay process, the exercise intensity of sport-specific ball drills could be targeted on the average or on the peak match demands across different time windows (Riboli et al. 2021e), as previously suggested (Taberner et al. 2019).

Nowadays, various aspects of load can be readily quantified by the GPS, gyroscopes, and accelerometers and offer an interesting opportunity to benchmark performance levels, quantify load and performance, and set sport-specific targets for RTSport. The decision-making process for RTPlay is an assessment based on a judgement of "functionality" and "performance capacity" rather than "clinical-functional suitability" (Bisciotti et al. 2019). The GPS technology was considered sufficient to inform objective criteria for RTPlay (Ardern et al. 2016; Bisciotti et al. 2019; Taberner et al. 2019; van der Horst et al. 2017; Zambaldi et al. 2017). The GPS tracking systems were considered an important tool for functional assessment by the majority of the experts due to their ability to mimic sport-specific function (van der Horst et al. 2017).

7.3 The Use of Imaging on the RTPlay Process

Basic science studies on muscle healing affirm that athletes are often allowed to return to play when the injured structures are not yet mature (Wangensteen et al. 2016). At the average moment of RTPlay, the muscle healing process is ongoing and scar tissue is still immature, leading to unremittingly high reoccurrences of reinjuries (Wangensteen et al. 2016). However, no strong evidence for the magnetic resonance imaging (MRI) findings that can guide sports physicians and radiologists in predicting prognosis for the time to RTPlay after muscle injuries seems currently available (Reurink et al. 2015a; van der Horst et al. 2017; van Heumen et al. 2017). There are only moderate evidences that injuries without hyperintensity on fluid-sensitive sequences are associated with a shorter time to RTPlay and that injuries involving the proximal free tendon are associated with a longer time to RTPlay (Reurink et al. 2015b). No strong current evidence for the association of any MRI finding at baseline and/or RTPlay with muscle reinjury was also reported (van Heumen et al. 2017). Connective tissue scar (fibrosis) is a common finding on MRI after recovery from acute muscle injuries and it has been suggested as a predisposing factor for reinjury (Reurink et al. 2015a). However, no evidence of the association between fibrosis assessment with MRI and reinjury is currently reported (Reurink et al. 2015a). On these bases, no consensus was gained by a worldwide expert panel on the use of MRI in the RTPlay process suggesting that MRI findings should not be used for RTPlay readiness assessment (van der Horst et al. 2017). Therefore, a comprehensive RTPlay functional test battery with adherence to the natural healing process of the injured tissue was recommended (Pieters et al. 2021). Before deciding RTPlay readiness, clinicians should reflect whether or not it is biologically possible for the injured tissue to have regained enough strength to withstand the sport-specific forces. In an attempt to reduce the detrimental injury–reinjury cycle, several authors suggested to consider subjectively a possible timeframe useful for biological healing (Pieters et al. 2021). Therefore, stakeholders should be aware to an unclear consensus about the use of imaging to assist the RTPlay process.

7.4 The Rehabilitation Process in the Gym

The early rehabilitation phases are characterized by physio care and gym-based physical preparation. The gym-based preparation may move from isometric exercises to sprinting activities through both bilateral and unilateral strength exercise with overweight (e.g., squat, split squat, hip trust, etc.). Early isometric exercises provide cyclic high-strain magnitudes postulated to increase tendon/aponeurosis stiffness, reduce tendon/aponeurosis strain, and enhance force development (Taberner et al. 2020). After that, dynamic exercises on isolated muscles and full range of motion exercises such as unloaded squats, split squats, etc. would improve morphological and neural factors, muscle and tendon strength, motor unit recruitment and synchronization, etc. (Suchomel et al. 2018; Taberner et al. 2020). Increases in load, velocity and more complex exercises using both loaded and unloaded exercises would prepare the athletes to the last part of gym-based training in which a full range of motion exercises with overweight, eccentric, and plyometric activities are required. The athletes' feelings, the recovery of such neuromuscular capacities, and the possibilities to perform low-intensity running exercises lead practitioners on the next rehabilitation steps. To overcome from a phase to the next one, a < 10% in peak force and power during isometric exercises (i.e., testing on force plates) between injured and uninjured body parts is a crucial issue. Depending on the injury type and severity, both isometric and dynamic strength and power testing with the aims to compare injury and uninjured body parts should accompany the decision-making process. Moreover, individual observations may have to be compared with the individual preinjury level. The latter are fundamental bases for training load management and exercise prescriptions. Over the rehabilitation process, the strength, power, and plyometric exercises may progress from bilateral to unilateral with a contextual increase in the multiple joint and plain activities. It should not be forgotten that higher strength abilities could reduce the likelihood of reinjury risk (McCall et al. 2020; Silva et al. 2015).

In this phase, cardiovascular and metabolic capacities should be developed using cycling or arm ergometers depending on the injury type; also running activities in antigravity conditions should accompany gym-based exercises to prepare athletes to more running-specific demands. On the next rehabilitation phases on the pitch, running-based exercises are required for the player to cope with more demanding running exercises.

7.5 The Rehabilitation Process on the Pitch

Nowadays, it is possible to gain objective information about on-pitch training load management before and after RTPlay. The monitoring of external load (e.g., GPS, local positioning systems, etc.), internal load (e.g., heart rate, etc.), and perceived load (e.g., rating of perceived exertion) metrics and athletes' self-report measures (i.e., quality of wellness, stress, sleep, recovery, pain, etc.; Thorpe et al. 2017) are valid and reliable tools to measure the psychophysiological and locomotor load imposed on each player. These metrics were suggested to manage safely the exercise prescriptions across the rehabilitation process (Ardern et al. 2016; Bisciotti et al. 2019; Taberner et al. 2019; van der Horst et al. 2017; Zambaldi et al. 2017). The GPS variables were reported as crucial to monitor the performance development and to recreate locomotor loads near to the competition demands. For these purposes, both average (Riboli et al. 2020) and maximal (Riboli et al. 2021e) official match requirements could be utilized as a reference for training prescriptions across different time windows.

Recent investigations (Allen et al. 2021; Taberner et al. 2019; Taberner and Cohen 2018) provided insights about the progression of perceptual and reactive neurocognitive challenges on the pitch using monitoring tools (i.e., GPS). Taberner et al. (2019) defined a five-phase framework in which a progressive control to chaos approach in training prescriptions was proposed:

1. Phase 1—high control: A gradual increase in the volume of linear running at lower speeds, thereby limiting high-speed running exposure (<60% maximal speed) and musculoskeletal demands. Minimize acceleration/deceleration and movement variability with the ball. To build player confidence.

2. Phase 2—moderate control: Progressively increase distance covered accelerating/decelerating (i.e., from 2 to 4 ms^2) relative to the player's preinjury training demands. Increase linear high-speed running (60–70% maximal speed) and change of direction activities with and without the ball increasing movement variability.
3. Phase 3—control to chaos: Introduce specific weekly structure to overload game components using football-specific drills. The musculoskeletal system should be adapted to specific energy systems through acceleration, deceleration, change of direction components, and high-speed running (>65–80% maximal speed).
4. Phase 4—moderate chaos: High-speed running (>75% maximal speed) increases further under both control and chaotic conditions. Sprint distance based on the player's relative match demands should be increased. The accumulated weekly distance should mimic the typical preinjury training levels.
5. Phase 5—high chaos: In the final phase, both average and peak position-specific official match demands should be replicated and/or overloaded without restrictions. The accumulated weekly distance and the training intensity should mimic the typical preinjury training levels and it should be organized accordingly to the team's weekly training load.

In the rehabilitation process, coaches and performance scientists should assess the individual cardiorespiratory (Riboli et al. 2022a) and strength/power (Barker et al. 2018) capacities to detect continuously the possible differences with preinjury levels and individual progression over time (Ardern et al. 2016; Bisciotti et al. 2019; Dunlop et al. 2020). The effectiveness of the physiological adaptation should be objectively determined across the training routine using both maximal or submaximal testing modalities (Riboli et al. 2021a, d). A full expert consensus (i.e., 100%) stated that the functional and performance assessment should achieve differences <10% than preinjury capacities; concurrently, a great consensus (i.e., ~94%) was gained to no pain or discomfort within the latest phases of the rehabilitation process (Dunlop et al. 2020; van der Horst et al. 2017; Zambaldi et al. 2017). Additionally, the acute weekly training load (e.g., internal and external loads including training and match demands) should achieve the preinjury workload through football-specific unpredicted movements. The simulation of official position-specific match demands both for average (Riboli et al. 2020) and peak demands (Oliva-Lozano et al. 2020; Riboli et al. 2021e) across training routine was previously stated as fundamental in the RTPlay process (Bisciotti et al. 2019; van der Horst et al. 2017; Zambaldi et al. 2017). Moreover, the achievement of repeated maximal individual sprinting speed without pain and/or discomfort was reported as a crucial issue for full training participation. The very-high-speed and sprint (i.e., ~100% maximal speed) running distance should be recreated using both individual position-specific ball drills and/or small-sided games in a specific area per player (Riboli et al. 2020, 2021c) progressing from a participation as "floater" (spare player) to an increase interaction with other players (Allen et al. 2021). Therefore, sprinting and high-speed running may be integrated into practice and targeted on 100% of worst-case match demands (e.g., volume, intensity) and on individual maximum speeds

(McCall et al. 2020). Using small-sided games, an area per player of ~300 m^2 player, ~200 m^2 player, or ~ 250 m^2 player could be utilized to replicate official match demands in adult (Riboli et al. 2020), U19 to U17, and U16 to U15 elite soccer players, respectively (Riboli et al. 2021c). However, a relative area per player similar to official match demands (i.e., ~350 m^2 player) is required to replicate the 4-min match-derived maximal intensities using small-sided games (Riboli et al. 2022b). Moreover, the distribution of the time spent at a different percentage than peak demands can be used as a possible reference to recreate or to overload such sport-specific metrics (Riboli et al. 2021b). For example, it was previously reported that 6 min at intensity higher than 80% of the 1-min peak demand for the distance >20 km h^{-1} could be used as a minimal reference to plan at least six repetitions of 1 min using soccer-specific positional drills during practice (Riboli et al. 2021b). Lastly, the player should cope well with the chronic adaptation to the high-intensity workload during full training participation without restrictions (Allen et al. 2021; Taberner et al. 2020).

7.6 Conclusions

An optimal RTPlay should aim to return the player in the shortest and safest time-frame considering all the information to reduce possibly the reinjury risks. A safe RTPlay decision-making process should consider several physical, physiological, and psychological quantitative and qualitative factors across the timeframe. Multiple stakeholders should be involved in the RTPlay decision-making process including the individual player, the sports medicine, the coaching, and the performance teams. A too quick RTPlay may result in pain, joint effusion, and/or minor injury and ultimately delay the full training participation and the return to competition. The benefit of a progressive RTPlay moving from low-intensity running to peak performance demands may increase the likelihood of a safe return to competition.

References

Akenhead R, Harley JA, Tweddle SP (2016) Examining the external training load of an English premier league football team with special reference to acceleration. J Strength Cond Res 30(9):2424–2432. https://doi.org/10.1519/JSC.0000000000001343

Allen T, Wilson S, Cohen DD, Taberner M (2021) Drill design using the 'control-chaos continuum': blending science and art during return to sport following knee injury in elite football. Phys Ther Sport 50:22–35. https://doi.org/10.1016/j.ptsp.2021.02.011

Andersen TE, Tenga A, Engebretsen L, Bahr R (2004) Video analysis of injuries and incidents in Norwegian professional football. Br J Sports Med 38(5):626–631. https://doi.org/10.1136/bjsm.2003.007955

Ardern CL, Glasgow P, Schneiders A, Witvrouw E, Clarsen B, Cools A, Gojanovic B, Griffin S, Khan KM, Moksnes H, Mutch SA, Phillips N, Reurink G, Sadler R, Silbernagel KG, Thorborg K, Wangensteen A, Wilk KE, Bizzini M (2016) 2016 consensus statement on return to sport from the first world congress in sports physical therapy, Bern. Br J Sports Med 50(14):853–864. https://doi.org/10.1136/bjsports-2016-096278

Barker LA, Harry JR, Mercer JA (2018) Relationships between countermovement jump ground reaction forces and jump height, reactive strength index, and jump time. J Strength Cond Res 32(1):248–254. https://doi.org/10.1519/JSC.0000000000002160

Bisciotti GN, Volpi P, Alberti G, Aprato A, Artina M, Auci A, Bait C, Belli A, Bellistri G, Bettinsoli P, Bisciotti A, Bisciotti A, Bona S, Bresciani M, Bruzzone A, Buda R, Buffoli M, Callini M, Canata G, Cardinali D, Chamari K (2019) Italian consensus statement (2020) on return to play after lower limb muscle injury in football (soccer). BMJ Open Sport Exerc Med 5(1):e000505. https://doi.org/10.1136/bmjsem-2018-00050

Castillo D, Raya-González J, Weston M, Yanci J (2021) Distribution of external load during acquisition training sessions and match play of a professional soccer team. J Strength Cond Res 35(12):3453–3458. https://doi.org/10.1519/JSC.0000000000003363

Dunlop G, Ardern CL, Andersen TE, Lewin C, Dupont G, Ashworth B, O'Driscoll G, Rolls A, Brown S, McCall A (2020) Return-to-play practices following hamstring injury: a worldwide survey of 131 premier league football teams. Sports Med 50(4):829–840. https://doi.org/10.1007/s40279-019-01199-2

Eirale C, Hamilton B, Bisciotti G, Grantham J, Chalabi H (2012) Injury epidemiology in a national football team of the Middle East. Scand J Med Sci Sports 22(3):323–329. https://doi.org/10.1111/j.1600-0838.2010.01227.x

Eirale C, Tol JL, Farooq A, Smiley F, Chalabi H (2013) Low injury rate strongly correlates with team success in Qatari professional football. Br J Sports Med 47(12):807–808. https://doi.org/10.1136/bjsports-2012-091040

Eirale C, Gillogly S, Singh G, Chamari K (2017) Injury and illness epidemiology in soccer—effects of global geographical differences—a call for standardized and consistent research studies. Biol Sport 34(3):249–254. https://doi.org/10.5114/biolsport.2017.66002

Ekstrand J (2013) Keeping your top players on the pitch: the key to football medicine at a professional level. Br J Sports Med 47(12):723–724. https://doi.org/10.1136/bjsports-2013-092771

Ekstrand J, Hägglund M, Waldén M (2011a) Epidemiology of muscle injuries in professional football (soccer). Am J Sports Med 39(6):1226–1232. https://doi.org/10.1177/0363546510395879

Ekstrand J, Hägglund M, Waldén M (2011b) Injury incidence and injury patterns in professional football: the UEFA injury study. Br J Sports Med 45(7):553–558. https://doi.org/10.1136/bjsm.2009.060582

Ekstrand J, Waldén M, Hägglund M (2016) Hamstring injuries have increased by 4% annually in men's professional football, since 2001: a 13-year longitudinal analysis of the UEFA elite club injury study. Br J Sports Med 50(12):731–737. https://doi.org/10.1136/bjsports-2015-095359

Gabbett TJ (2016) The training-injury prevention paradox: should athletes be training smarter and harder? Br J Sports Med 50(5):273–280. https://doi.org/10.1136/bjsports-2015-095788

Gregson W, Di Salvo V, Varley MC, Modonutti M, Belli A, Chamari K, Weston M, Lolli L, Eirale C (2020) Harmful association of sprinting with muscle injury occurrence in professional soccer match-play: a two-season, league wide exploratory investigation from the Qatar stars league. J Sci Med Sport 23(2):134–138. https://doi.org/10.1016/j.jsams.2019.08.289

Hägglund M, Waldén M, Magnusson H, Kristenson K, Bengtsson H, Ekstrand J (2013) Injuries affect team performance negatively in professional football: an 11-year follow-up of the UEFA champions league injury study. Br J Sports Med 47(12):738–742. https://doi.org/10.1136/bjsports-2013-092215

Hawkins RD, Fuller CW (1999) A prospective epidemiological study of injuries in four English professional football clubs. Br J Sports Med 33(3):196–203. https://doi.org/10.1136/bjsm.33.3.196

Hawkins RD, Hulse MA, Wilkinson C, Hodson A, Gibson M (2001) The association football medical research programme: an audit of injuries in professional football. Br J Sports Med 35(1):43–47. https://doi.org/10.1136/bjsm.35.1.43

Herring SA, Kibler WB, Putukian M (2012) The team physician and the return-to-play decision: a consensus statement-2012 update. Med Sci Sports Exerc 44(12):2446–2448. https://doi.org/10.1249/MSS.0b013e3182750534

Herring SA, Kibler WB, Putukian M (2013) Team physician consensus statement: 2013 update. Med Sci Sports Exerc 45(8):1618–1622. https://doi.org/10.1249/MSS.0b013e31829ba437

Lacome M, Simpson BM, Cholley Y, Lambert P, Buchheit M (2018) Small-sided games in elite soccer: does one size fit all? Int J Sports Physiol Perform 13(5):568–576. https://doi.org/10.1123/ijspp.2017-021

Lauersen JB, Andersen TE, Andersen LB (2018) Strength training as superior, dose-dependent and safe prevention of acute and overuse sports injuries: a systematic review, qualitative analysis and meta-analysis. Br J Sports Med 52(24):1557–1563. https://doi.org/10.1136/bjsports-2018-099078

Le Gall F, Carling C, Reilly T, Vandewalle H, Church J, Rochcongar P (2006) Incidence of injuries in elite French youth soccer players: a 10-season study. Am J Sports Med 34(6):928–938. https://doi.org/10.1177/0363546505283271

Martín-García A, Gómez Díaz A, Bradley PS, Morera F, Casamichana D (2018) Quantification of a professional football team's external load using a microcycle structure. J Strength Cond Res 32(12):3511–3518. https://doi.org/10.1519/JSC.0000000000002816

McCall A, Pruna R, Van der Horst N, Dupont G, Buchheit M, Coutts AJ, Impellizzeri FM, Fanchini M, EFP-Group (2020) Exercise-based strategies to prevent muscle injury in male elite footballers: an expert-led Delphi survey of 21 practitioners belonging to 18 teams from the big-5 European Leagues. Sports Med 50(9):1667–1681. https://doi.org/10.1007/s40279-020-01315-7

Morgan BE, Oberlander MA (2001) An examination of injuries in major league soccer. The inaugural season. Am J Sports Med 29(4):426–430. https://doi.org/10.1177/03635465010290040701

Oliva-Lozano JM, Rojas-Valverde D, Gómez-Carmona CD, Fortes V, Pino-Ortega J (2020) Worst case scenario match analysis and contextual variables in professional soccer players: a longitudinal study. Biol Sport 37(4):429–436. https://doi.org/10.5114/biolsport.2020.97067

Orchard JW (2009) On the value of team medical staff: can the "Moneyball" approach be applied to injuries in professional football? Br J Sports Med 43(13):963–965. https://doi.org/10.1136/bjsm.2009.05840

Pfirrmann D, Herbst M, Ingelfinger P, Simon P, Tug S (2016) Analysis of injury incidences in male professional adult and elite youth soccer players: a systematic review. J Athl Train 51(5):410–424. https://doi.org/10.4085/1062-6050-51.6.03

Pieters D, Wezenbeek E, Schuermans J, Witvrouw E (2021) Return to play after a hamstring strain injury: it is time to consider natural healing. Sports Med 51(10):2067–2077. https://doi.org/10.1007/s40279-021-01494-x

Price RJ, Hawkins RD, Hulse MA, Hodson A (2004) The football association medical research programme: an audit of injuries in academy youth football. Br J Sports Med 38(4):466–471. https://doi.org/10.1136/bjsm.2003.005165

Reurink G, Almusa E, Goudswaard GJ, Tol JL, Hamilton B, Moen MH, Weir A, Verhaar JA, Maas M (2015a) No association between fibrosis on magnetic resonance imaging at return to play and hamstring reinjury risk. Am J Sports Med 43(5):1228–1234. https://doi.org/10.1177/0363546515572603

Reurink G, Brilman EG, de Vos RJ, Maas M, Moen MH, Weir A, Goudswaard GJ, Tol JL (2015b) Magnetic resonance imaging in acute hamstring injury: can we provide a return to play prognosis? Sports Med 45(1):133–146. https://doi.org/10.1007/s40279-014-0243-

Riboli A, Coratella G, Rampichini S, Cé E, Esposito F (2020) Area per player in small-sided games to replicate the external load and estimated physiological match demands in elite soccer players. PLoS One 15(9):e0229194. https://doi.org/10.1371/journal.pone.0229194

Riboli A, Dellal A, Esposito F, Coratella G (2021a) Can small-sided games assess the training-induced aerobic adaptations in elite football players? J Sports Med Phys Fitness 62(10):1313. https://doi.org/10.23736/S0022-4707.21.13144-5; Advance online publication

Riboli A, Esposito F, Coratella G (2021b) The distribution of match activities relative to the maximal intensities in elite soccer players: implications for practice. Res Sports Med 30(5):463. https://doi.org/10.1080/15438627.2021.1895788; Advance online publication

Riboli A, Olthof SB, Esposito F, Coratella G (2021c) Training elite youth soccer players: area per player in small-sided games to replicate the match demands. Biol Sport 39(3):579–598. https://doi.org/10.5114/biolsport.2022.106388

Riboli A, Rampichini S, Cè E, Limonta E, Borrelli M, Coratella G, Esposito F (2021d) Training status affects between-protocols differences in the assessment of maximal aerobic velocity. Eur J Appl Physiol 121(11):3083–3093. https://doi.org/10.1007/s00421-021-04763-9

Riboli A, Semeria M, Coratella G, Esposito F (2021e) Effect of formation, ball in play and ball possession on peak demands in elite soccer. Biol Sport 38(2):195–205. https://doi.org/10.5114/biolsport.2020.98450

Riboli A, Coratella G, Rampichini S, Limonta E, Esposito F (2022a) Testing protocol affects the velocity at VO2max in semi-professional soccer players. Res Sports Med 30(2):182–192. https://doi.org/10.1080/15438627.2021.1878460

Riboli A, Esposito F, Coratella G (2022b) Small-sided games in elite football: practical solutions to replicate the 4-min match-derived maximal intensities. J Strength Cond Res 37:366. https://doi.org/10.1519/JSC.0000000000004249; Advance online publication

Ritchie D, Hopkins WG, Buchheit M, Cordy J, Bartlett JD (2017) Quantification of training load during return to play after upper- and lower-body injury in Australian rules football. Int J Sports Physiol Perform 12(5):634–641. https://doi.org/10.1123/ijspp.2016-0300

Silva JR, Nassis GP, Rebelo A (2015) Strength training in soccer with a specific focus on highly trained players. Sports Med Open 1(1):17. https://doi.org/10.1186/s40798-015-0006-z

Stevens TG, de Ruiter CJ, Twisk JW, Savelsbergh GJ, Beek PJ (2017) Quantification of in-season training load relative to match load in professional Dutch Eredivisie football players. Sci Med Footb 1(2):117–125. https://doi.org/10.1080/24733938.2017.1282163

Suchomel TJ, Nimphius S, Bellon CR, Stone MH (2018) The importance of muscular strength: training considerations. Sports Med 48(4):765–785. https://doi.org/10.1007/s40279-018-0862-z

Taberner M, Cohen DD (2018) Physical preparation of the football player with an intramuscular hamstring tendon tear: clinical perspective with video demonstrations. Br J Sports Med 52(19):1275–1278. https://doi.org/10.1136/bjsports-2017-098817

Taberner M, Allen T, Cohen DD (2019) Progressing rehabilitation after injury: consider the 'control-chaos continuum'. Br J Sports Med 53(18):1132–1136. https://doi.org/10.1136/bjsports-2018-100157

Taberner M, van Dyk N, Allen T, Jain N, Richter C, Drust B, Betancur E, Cohen DD (2020) Physical preparation and return to performance of an elite female football player following ACL reconstruction: a journey to the FIFA Women's world cup. BMJ Open Sport Exerc Med 6(1):e000843. https://doi.org/10.1136/bmjsem-2020-000843

Thorpe RT, Atkinson G, Drust B, Gregson W (2017) Monitoring fatigue status in elite team-sport athletes: implications for practice. Int J Sports Physiol Perform 12(Suppl 2):S227–S234. https://doi.org/10.1123/ijspp.2016-0434

van der Horst N, Backx F, Goedhart EA, Huisstede BM, HIPS-Delphi Group (2017) Return to play after hamstring injuries in football (soccer): a worldwide Delphi procedure regarding definition, medical criteria and decision-making. Br J Sports Med 51(22):1583–1591. https://doi.org/10.1136/bjsports-2016-097206

van Heumen M, Tol JL, de Vos RJ, Moen MH, Weir A, Orchard J, Reurink G (2017) The prognostic value of MRI in determining reinjury risk following acute hamstring injury: a systematic review. Br J Sports Med 51(18):1355–1363. https://doi.org/10.1136/bjsports-2016-096790

Waldén M, Hägglund M, Ekstrand J (2005) UEFA champions league study: a prospective study of injuries in professional football during the 2001-2002 season. Br J Sports Med 39(8):542–546. https://doi.org/10.1136/bjsm.2004.014571

Wangensteen A, Tol JL, Witvrouw E, Van Linschoten R, Almusa E, Hamilton B, Bahr R (2016) Hamstring reinjuries occur at the same location and early after return to sport: a descriptive study of MRI-confirmed reinjuries. Am J Sports Med 44(8):2112–2121. https://doi.org/10.1177/0363546516646086

Yoon YS, Chai M, Shin DW (2004) Football injuries at Asian tournaments. Am J Sports Med 32(1 Suppl):36S–42S. https://doi.org/10.1177/0095399703258781

Zambaldi M, Beasley I, Rushton A (2017) Return to play criteria after hamstring muscle injury in professional football: a Delphi consensus study. Br J Sports Med 51(16):1221–1226. https://doi.org/10.1136/bjsports-2016-097131

Manipulation and Delivery of Training Load Into a Seasonal Schedule

8

Hadi Nobari and Rafael Oliveira

Training load monitoring has become a mandatory practice in professional and non-professional soccer. The aim of this chapter was to describe the common practices on the manipulation of the training load and how to deliver a better intensity in a season schedule. To accomplish these aims, this chapter described information on periodization concepts and practical example on the load applied during mesocycles and microcycles with one, two, and three matches. The information of this chapter contextualized that mesocycles from preseason and from the beginning of the season (first three mesocycles) provided higher load when compared with the remaining mesocycles of the season. Considering data from microcycles, matches revealed to be the days with the highest intensity, being followed by training sessions of middle days of the week. Specifically, higher load was found between 5 and 3 days before the match, while the lowest values were found on the day before the match.

This chapter intends to present information on how to organize different seasonal schedules for weeks with one match or congested weeks (i.e., more than one match per week). The topic about training load is frequent and constitutes a daily practice in professional clubs (Weston 2018). Recently, the term "load" was discussed and its replacement with the term "intensity" was suggested by the "International System of Units" (Staunton et al. 2021). To avoid confusion to the readers, "training load" was used in this chapter according to a significant number of research, although intensity may be a better definition.

H. Nobari (✉)
Faculty of Sport Sciences, University of Extremadura, Cáceres, Spain

R. Oliveira
Sports Science School of Rio Maior–Polytechnic Institute of Santarém, Rio Maior, Portugal

Research Centre in Sport Sciences, Health Sciences and Human Development, Vila Real, Portugal

J. M. Oliva Lozano, L. P. Ardigò (eds.), *Training Load in Professional Soccer*,
https://doi.org/10.1007/978-3-031-52087-7_8

One of the biggest challenges for coaches is the design of training programs to induce optimal training adaptations and maximize performance at the desired instants of the competitive season (Mujika et al. 2018). Depending on the level of the competition and team, soccer players should be prepared to complete between 3 and 7 training sessions per week and compete once or twice a week during the competition period (i.e., for 9–10 months of a domestic league). Although some high-level soccer teams often experience congested calendars, most young, amateur, and professional soccer teams usually have to play one match per week. However, the organization of the weekly training load should warrant peak performance in the most important session of the week, which is the official match, regardless of the competition level and match fixtures (Rico-González et al. 2020).

Soccer is continually evolving and this requires coaches to design training protocols with different periodization strategies that optimize physical and technical adaptations (Fessi et al. 2016a, b; Kelly et al. 2020; Moalla et al. 2016). However, weekly soccer training programs differ according to the phase of the annual plan, the number of season weeks, and/or the experience of the coach as mentioned before (Bangsbo et al. 2006). Training plans are usually divided into mesocycles. Each mesocycle is generally divided into 3 to 5 microcycles, which have a specific training goal that ultimately focuses on the final performance target (Gamble 2006; Jeong et al. 2011; Mujika et al. 2018). To achieve optimal performance on match day, Gamble's approach suggests a variation of each summated microcycle duration according to the schedule of competitive matches (Gamble 2006). Consequently, coaches must find a balance between training stimulus and recovery to optimize physiological adaptations and performance. Indeed, most coaches carry out a short-term reduction of training load, usually at the end of each mesocycle block (Fessi et al. 2016a, b). This short-term progressive reduction of training load is called "tapering" and is intended to decrease fatigue caused by training and to optimize physiological and psychological adaptations before a competition (Moalla et al. 2021).

With such different scenarios and variables to manipulate, it is extremely important to understand the training periodization strategies applied to soccer teams. Therefore, the aim of this chapter is to present training periodization conceptualization and training load periodization strategies for regular competitive schedules and congested calendars.

8.1 Training Periodization

The concept of periodization is a common topic of discussion among coaches and sports scientists. Classically, periodization can be divided into three levels: the macrocycle (long length, lasting 3–4 months), the mesocycle (mid-length, lasting 2–4 weeks), and the microcycle (short length, lasting 1–7 days). Each macrocycle generally begins with a format of high-volume, low-intensity training and ends with a reverse format of high-intensity, low-volume training (Bompa and Haff 2009; Matveyev 1981; Plisk and Stone 2003). In general, the macrocycle comprises four phases: preparation (general and special), competition, peaking, and transition or active rest. All these phases have different goals and degrees of variation.

However, classic periodization is somewhat difficult to put into practice during soccer trainings because it is essential that the team is well prepared for the game every week. For instance, top European players usually participate in 1–2 training sessions between two consecutive matches. For this reason and in this case, coaches can only implement recovery training (Akenhead et al. 2016; Anderson et al. 2016a, b; Malone et al. 2015; Stevens et al. 2017).

According to a previous study, the periodization plan for team sports could be divided in the following phases (Mujika et al. 2018):

- General preparation.
- Specific preparation, which is also known as pre-competition.
- Main competition or regular season.
- Playoffs or finals.
- Transition/off-season/injury.

When applied to soccer, general and specific preparations are associated to the preseason period where strength and conditioning capacities are developed in the beginning, and a higher intensity is then applied along with soccer-friendly matches. Then, the players get into the main competition or regular season, in which training and official matches occur. Playoffs or finals may also belong to this period (it depends on the level of the soccer team and the competitions the team belong). Finally, the last period is known as off-season for an active and passive recovery of the players. Thus, training load needs to be monitored during these phases.

8.2 Microcycle Periodization

One of the first studies that analyzed seasonal training load data from soccer players during a full season was published in 2015 (Malone et al. 2015). These authors analyzed English Premier League players in weeks with one match during pre- and in-season periods (Malone et al. 2015). The study analyzed microcycles with four training sessions, namely, MD−5, 5 days before the match; MD−3, 3 days before the match; MD−2, 2 days before the match; and MD−1, the day before the match. MD−4 and the day after the match (MD + 1) were days off. The day after the match. The authors found that MD−1 was the day with the lowest load while the other days presented similar values in variables such as total distance, high-speed running distance, and session RPE. There was a few load variation across the typical microcycle over the season. The authors also found positional differences regarding the load applied (Malone et al. 2015) which should be considered when preparing training periodization for the entire team.

Recently, a similar study with Elite Portuguese Premier League soccer players (Oliveira et al. 2019b) analyzed 10 in-season mesocycles and the most typical microcycle for weeks with only one match of the in-season period. It was concluded that despite the existence of some significant differences between mesocycles, there were minor changes across the in-season period (a tendency of higher values in the first three mesocycles of the in-season was observed) for internal and external training load (e.g., total distance, high-speed running, or session RPE) and perceived wellness, which was collected through the Hooper index. Furthermore, a microcycle pattern showed that MD−1 presented a general reduction of training load while the other days kept a similar training intensity. In addition, Hooper index variables only showed significant differences in the day after the match where higher values were revealed, while the other days remained identical.

Even more recently, a study analyzed the effect of the length of the microcycle across a full season in La Liga 123 (Oliva-Lozano et al. 2022). In this study, short (five training sessions), regular (six training sessions), and long microcycles (seven training sessions) were considered. The study found that the highest intensity and volume were found to be on match day, being followed by MD−4 and MD−3 for total distance covered, total number of high-intensity accelerations and decelerations, total number of high-speed running actions, high-speed running distance, and player load regardless of the microcycle length. Intrinsically, this study showed the lowest values on MD−2 (but the values were similar to MD−1) regardless of the microcycle length. Finally, when comparing data from different microcycles, a significant effect on all variables were found with the exception for high-intensity accelerations and decelerations and high metabolic load distance (Oliva-Lozano et al. 2022). In the same line with the previous studies, other studies considered the worst-case scenario analysis (the most demanding passages, which are considered the most intense periods of a match or training) and found the same results (Oliva-Lozano et al. 2021).

In line with the previous information is a systematic review (in press) that found a post-match recovery strategy followed by an increase in intensity until MD−3 and MD−2 (Cano et al. 2022). The same study added that microcycles with more matches per week presented a higher focus on recovery, meaning a decrease in intensity through the microcycle. During the 2 matches' week, a lower intensity or one recovery day is suggested after the match. Meanwhile, in the 3 matches' week, coaches should prescribe recovery sessions in the days between matches (Cano et al. 2022).

Considering weeks with one match, coaches should program the training with a higher load between MD−5 and MD−3 (50–75% (<52 m/min) of the match distance covered, between 25% and 72% of match high-speed running covered (< 25 m/min), and between 57% and 92% of the total accelerations performed during the competition. Moreover, weeks with two matches present a similar pattern of weeks with one match. For the most intense sessions (MD−3 and MD−2), a total distance covered between 60% and 66% of the match independently of the microcycle length, between 15% and 39% of the match high-intensity running covered, and between 3% and 19% at sprint distance covered. Finally, in weeks with three matches, the intensity should be reduced for maintaining between 51% and 98% of total distance covered at low intensity during competition (Cano et al. 2022).

A general consensus that match day is the day with higher load was shown to be in line with several studies (Bradley et al. 2009; Los et al. 2017; Los Arcos et al.

2014; Malone et al. 2015; Oliva-Lozano et al. 2022; Oliveira et al. 2019a, b; Stevens et al. 2017). The reasons that explained the results were associated with the need to win matches that obliged coaches to reduce load when MD was near (i.e., MD−1) (Malone et al. 2015; Oliveira et al. 2019b), in order to avoid injuries and illness (Akenhead et al. 2016; Fessi et al. 2016a, b; Jeong et al. 2011; Malone et al. 2015).

Moreover, a systematic review about in-season weekly training load for weeks with one match showed that training load that came from the match represented 38% of the weekly differentiated session RPE, being almost the exclusive source of weekly high-speed and sprinting (90–97%) in professional soccer players. It was also found that the number of weekly training sessions carried out by the team does not seem to influence weekly training load in both professional and young soccer players. Training load progressively increased up to 4 days after the previous match (i.e., 3 days before the next match) to get reduced up to the day before the competition in professional soccer players, but a clear trend for weekly training load distribution was not apparent for young soccer players (Rico-González et al. 2020).

Furthermore, two recent systematic reviews summarized information on training intensity in young (Oliveira et al. 2021c) and professional soccer players (Oliveira et al. 2022). Similar to the previous reports, both studies confirmed the lowest intensity on MD−1 considering external and internal measures. In young soccer players, this finding was evident between under-15 and under-19 categories (Oliveira et al. 2021c). Both studies found higher values in the middle days of the week (Oliveira et al. 2021a, 2022).

However, the complex nature of soccer competition and training complicates the individual prescription of the weekly training load, which results in considerable differences in training load between soccer players of the same team (Akubat et al. 2012), since there are different playing positions (Clemente et al. 2020; Oliveira et al. 2019b) and status (starters and nonstarters) (Nobari et al. 2020a, b, c, 2021a).

In a soccer match, only 11 players participate from the beginning of the match and only three could be replaced, which means the other players in the bench do not participate in the most demanding session of the week (Los et al. 2017; Los Arcos et al. 2014). As a consequence, coaches apply compensatory training strategies, but several studies reported higher weekly training load for the starters when compared to nonstarters (Azcárate et al. 2018; Los et al. 2017; Nobari et al. 2020a, c, 2021a, b, c). In addition, strategical (e.g., playing system and positions) and situational variables (e.g., opponent's level, match location, and period of the season) (Nobari et al. 2021b; Oliveira et al. 2020, 2021a) can substantially influence training and match loads.

Regarding the microcycle training sessions, some studies (Anderson et al. 2016b; Los et al. 2017; Thorpe et al. 2016) found that coaches periodized training contents to attain the highest weekly training load in the middle of the week. Training load increased until 4 days following the previous match (i.e., 3 days before the next match) and later decreases up to the day before the competition (Los et al. 2017; Thorpe et al. 2016). As a result, an increasing-decreasing training load trend is suggested during the training week until the most demanding session of the week, the official match, in professional soccer players. Then, a recovery period needs to be applied to manage fatigue.

Therefore and according to previous research (Rico-González et al. 2020), professional soccer teams accumulate lower session RPE (1200–1600 AUs) for one-match young soccer players (2500–4000 AUs) during in-season period. Moreover, inter-player training, match, and weekly training load variability are greater for professional soccer players in comparison to young soccer players. Match participation is the main contributor of the one-match weekly training load (>32–36% of the total internal and external weekly training load) and almost the exclusive source of weekly high-speed and sprinting running in professional soccer players. However, the impact of the match on the one-match weekly training load is less clear in young soccer teams. It seems that the number of training sessions carried out by the teams during the week does not influence the global weekly training load in both professional and young soccer players. Training load progressively increased up to 4 days after the previous match (i.e., 3 days before the next match) to get reduced up to the day before the competition in professional soccer players, but a clear trend for weekly training load distribution along the week in young soccer players is not apparent.

8.3 Mesocycle Periodization

Since periodization includes more than one microcycle analyses across the entire season, it is relevant to acknowledge are the strategies for mesocycles. According to Coutts et al. (2008), coaches have been recommended to adopt effective recovery strategies between training sessions and impose a short-term reduction of training load at the end of every mesocycle. The reduction of training load is known as "tapering." In other words, tapering consists of reducing the physiological and psychological stress of training to maximize performance after an intense training period (Bosquet et al. 2007). Regarding microcycle training, it was observed that training load was reduced to MD−1, what could be considered as a tapering strategy (Anderson et al. 2016b; Los et al. 2017; Malone et al. 2015; Oliveira et al. 2019a, b, 2021b).

Basically, tapering could be characterized by a reduction of the training load volume and frequency. However, training intensity should be maintained during the taper period which can be achieved by performing high-intensity interval training (Bosquet et al. 2007).

In this regard, some authors (Fessi et al. 2016a, b) examined the effect of decreasing training load during taper weeks on physical match activities in professional soccer players. They concluded that decreasing training load by ~25% during taper weeks by reducing training duration and frequency but maintaining intensity was associated with a 15% increase in physical activities during matches.

On the other hand, a previous study analyzed 10 mesocycles of the in-season period. However, no such strategies were identified and the general conclusion showed that mesocycles were similar across the in-season with higher values being noted in the beginning of the in-season (mesocycles 1–3) (Oliveira et al. 2019b).

Two studies (Kelly et al. 2020; Malone et al. 2015) also examined training load quantification and its distribution throughout the season utilizing a periodization of six standard and equivalent mesocycles separated into 6 weeks. One study (Malone et al. 2015) found that the preseason training load showed limited variation across each microcycle, while the other study (Kelly et al. 2020) concluded that training load across the mesocycle periods showed limited variation and suggests that training schedules of elite soccer may be highly repetitive, likely reflecting the nature of the competition demands. However, a recent study highlighted that the duration of the mesocycle can influence changes in match running performance following a tapering period in soccer. The study showed no significant difference in the training load parameters or match running performance during matches within standard weeks. Meanwhile, match running performance following the taper weeks varied according to mesocycle duration, though the difference in training load parameters is not significant (Moalla et al. 2021). Consequently, the authors suggested that mesocycles of four microcycles should end with a tapering period (3 standard weeks with 1 tapering week), which depends on the match objectives to enhance physical activities, prevent acute fatigue and overtraining, and maintain match readiness. Therefore, soccer coaches should consider designing tapering weeks by decreasing the training frequency and duration while maintaining intensity compared to the previous training load already accomplished in pre-tapering to optimize match running performance, especially high-intensity activities (Moalla et al. 2021).

8.4 Recommendations for Future Studies

Indeed, there are a lot of literature in training load quantification with respect to soccer periodization strategies; however, the majority of the scientific evidence only presents the different internal and external measures applied (session RPE, heart rate, blood lactate, total distance, different speed thresholds, accelerations, deceleration, player load, metabolic power, etc.) as well as workload measures (training monotony, strain, and acute/chronic workload ratio). Therefore, this chapter recommends that future studies could analyze and explain what the training periodization strategies are applied with special regard to the different types of exercises that are applied. Only with such information, it will be possible to properly understand periodization strategies as well as to replicate studies.

References

Akenhead R, Harley JA, Tweddle SP (2016) Examining the external training load of an English premier league football team with special reference to acceleration. J Strength Cond Res 30(9):2424–2432. https://doi.org/10.1519/JSC.0000000000001343

Akubat I, Patel E, Barrett S, Abt G (2012) Methods of monitoring the training and match load and their relationship to changes in fitness in professional youth soccer players. J Sports Sci 30:1473–1480. https://doi.org/10.1080/02640414.2012.712711

Anderson L, Orme P, Di Michele R, Close GL, Milsom J, Morgans R, Drust B, Morton JP (2016a) Quantification of seasonal-long physical load in soccer players with different starting status from the English premier league: implications for maintaining squad physical fitness. Int J Sports Physiol Perform 11(8):1038–1046

Anderson L, Orme P, Di Michele R, Close GL, Morgans R, Drust B, Morton JP (2016b) Quantification of training load during one-, two- and three-game week schedules in professional soccer players from the English premier league: implications for carbohydrate periodisation. J Sports Sci 34(13):1250–1259. https://doi.org/10.1080/02640414.2015.1106574

Azcárate U, Yanci J, Los Arcos A (2018) Influence of match playing time and the length of the between-match microcycle in Spanish professional soccer players' perceived training load. Sci Med Footb 2:23–28

Bangsbo J, Mohr M, Krustrup P (2006) Physical and metabolic demands of training and match-play in the elite football player. J Sports Sci 24(7):665–674. https://doi.org/10.1080/02640410500482529

Bompa T, Haff G (2009) Periodization, theory and methodology of training, 5th edn. H. Kinetics

Bosquet L, Montpetit J, Arvisais D, Mujika I (2007) Effects of tapering on performance: a meta-analysis. Med Sci Sports Exerc 39(8):1358–1365. https://doi.org/10.1249/mss.0b013e31806010e0

Bradley PS, Sheldon W, Wooster B, Olsen P, Boanas P, Krustrup P (2009) High-intensity running in English FA premier league soccer matches. J Sports Sci 27:159–168. https://doi.org/10.1080/02640410802512775

Cano JR, Martín-García A, Rico González M (2022) Training intensity management during microcycles, mesocycles, and macrocycles in soccer: a systematic review. Proc Inst Mech Eng P J Sports Eng Technol; In press

Clemente FM, Silva R, Ramirez-Campillo R, Afonso J, Mendes B, Chen YS (2020) Accelerometry-based variables in professional soccer players: comparisons between periods of the season and playing positions. Biol Sport 37(4):389–403. https://doi.org/10.5114/BIOLSPORT.2020.96852

Coutts AJ, Chamari K, Impellizzeri FM, Rampinini E (2008) Monitoring training in soccer: measuring and periodising training. In: Alexandre D (ed) De l'entraînement à la performance en football [from training to performance in soccer], Bruxelles

Fessi MS, Zarrouk N, Di Salvo V, Filetti C, Barker AR, Moalla W (2016a) Effects of tapering on physical match activities in professional soccer players. J Sports Sci 34(24):2189–2194. https://doi.org/10.1080/02640414.2016.1171891

Fessi MS, Zarrouk N, Filetti C, Rebai H, Elloumi M, Moalla W (2016b) Physical and anthropometric changes during pre- and in-season in professional soccer players. J Sports Med Phys Fitness 56(10):1163–1170

Gamble P (2006) Periodization of training for team sports athletes. Strength Cond J 28(5):55–66. https://doi.org/10.1519/00126548-200610000-00009

Jeong TS, Reilly T, Morton J, Bae SW, Drust B (2011) Quantification of the physiological loading of one week of "pre-season" and one week of "in-season" training in professional soccer players. J Sports Sci 29(11):1161–1166. https://doi.org/10.1080/02640414.2011.583671; PubMed ID: 21777053

Kelly DM, Strudwick AJ, Atkinson G, Drust B, Gregson W (2020) Quantification of training and match-load distribution across a season in elite English premier league soccer players. Sci Med Footb 4(1):59–67. https://doi.org/10.1080/24733938.2019.1651934

Los Arcos A, Yanci J, Mendiguchia J, Gorostiaga EM (2014) Rating of muscular and respiratory perceived exertion in professional soccer players. J Strength Cond Res 28:3280–3288. https://doi.org/10.1519/JSC.0000000000000540

Los AA, Mendez-Villanueva A, Martínez-Santos R (2017) In-season training periodization of professional soccer players. Biol Sport 34(2):149–155. https://doi.org/10.5114/biolsport.2017.64588

Malone J, Di Michele R, Morgans R, Burgess D, Morton J, Drust B (2015) Seasonal training-load quantification in elite English premier league soccer players. Int J Sports Physiol Perform 10:489–497. https://doi.org/10.1123/ijspp.2014-0352

Matveyev L (1981) Fundamentals of sports training; (Progress P)
Moalla W, Fessi MS, Farhat F, Nouira S, Wong DP, Dupont G (2016) Relationship between daily training load and psychometric status of professional soccer players. Res Sports Med 24(4):387–394. https://doi.org/10.1080/15438627.2016.1239579
Moalla W, Fessi MS, Nouira S, Mendez-Villanueva A, Di Salvo V, Ahmaidi S (2021) Optimal pre-taper phase on physical match performance in professional soccer. Int J Sports Physiol Perform 1–7:1483. https://doi.org/10.1123/ijspp.2020-0334
Mujika I, Halson S, Burke LM, Balagué G, Farrow D (2018) An integrated, multifactorial approach to periodization for optimal performance in individual and team sports. Int J Sports Physiol Perform 13(5):538–561. https://doi.org/10.1123/ijspp.2018-0093
Nobari H, Aquino R, Clemente FM, Khalafi M, Adsuar JC, Pérez-Gómez J (2020a) Description of acute and chronic load, training monotony and strain over a season and its relationships with well-being status: a study in elite under-16 soccer players. Physiol Behav 225:113117. https://doi.org/10.1016/j.physbeh.2020.113117
Nobari H, Oliveira R, Clemente FM, Adsuar JC, Pérez-Gómez J, Carlos-Vivas J, Brito JP (2020b) Comparisons of accelerometer variables training monotony and strain of starters and non-starters: a full-season study in professional soccer players. Int J Environ Res Public Health 17(18):1–14. https://doi.org/10.3390/ijerph17186547
Nobari H, Praça GM, Clemente FM, Pérez-Gómez J, Carlos Vivas J, Ahmadi M (2020c) Comparisons of new body load and metabolic power average workload indices between starters and non-starters: a full-season study in professional soccer players. Proc Inst Mech Eng P J Sports Eng Technol 235:105. https://doi.org/10.1177/1754337120974873
Nobari H, Castillo D, Clemente FM, Carlos-Vivas J, Pérez-Gómez J (2021a) Acute, chronic and acute/chronic ratio between starters and non-starters professional soccer players across a competitive season. Proc Inst Mech Eng P J Sports Eng Technol 285:175433712110165. https://doi.org/10.1177/17543371211016594
Nobari H, Oliveira R, Jorge P, Clemente FM, Paolo L (2021b) Comparison of running distance variables and body load in competitions based on their results: a full-season study of professional soccer players. Int J Environ Res Public Health 18:2077
Nobari H, Vahabidelshad R, Pérez-Gómez J, Ardigò LP (2021c) Variations of training workload in micro- and meso-cycles based on position in elite young soccer players: a competition season study. Front Physiol 12(1):1–10. https://doi.org/10.3389/fphys.2021.668145
Oliva-Lozano JM, Gómez-Carmona CD, Rojas-Valverde D, Fortes V, Pino-Ortega J (2021) Effect of training day, match, and length of the microcycle on the worst-case scenarios in professional soccer players. Res Sports Med 1:1–14. https://doi.org/10.1080/15438627.2021.1895786
Oliva-Lozano JM, Gómez-Carmona CD, Fortes V, Pino-Ortega J (2022) Effect of training day, match, and length of the microcycle on workload periodization in professional soccer players: a full-season study. Biol Sport 39(2):397–406. https://doi.org/10.5114/biolsport.2022.106148
Oliveira R, Brito J, Martins A, Mendes B, Calvete F, Carriço S, Ferraz R, Marques MC (2019a) In-season training load quantification of one-, two- and three-game week schedules in a top European professional soccer team. Physiol Behav 201:146. https://doi.org/10.1016/j.physbeh.2018.11.036
Oliveira R, Brito JP, Martins A, Mendes B, Marinho DA, Ferraz R, Marques MC (2019b) In-season internal and external training load quantification of an elite European soccer team. PLoS One 14(4):e0209393. https://doi.org/10.1371/journal.pone.0209393
Oliveira R, Brito JP, Loureiro N, Padinha V, Ferreira B, Mendes B (2020) Does the distribution of the weekly training load account for the match results of elite professional soccer players? Physiol Behav 225:113118. https://doi.org/10.1016/j.physbeh.2020.113118
Oliveira R, Brito JP, Loureiro N, Padinha V, Nobari H, Mendes B (2021a) Will next match location influence external and internal training load of a top-class elite professional European soccer team? Int J Environ Res Public Health 18(10):5229. https://doi.org/10.3390/ijerph18105229
Oliveira R, Brito JM, Loureiro N, Padinha V, Ferreira B, Mendes B (2021b) Effects of match location, match result and the quality of opposition in training load on a two-matches week in a

top-class elite European soccer team Efectos de la ubicación del juego, el resultado del juego y la calidad del oponente, sobre la carga d. Cuadernos Psicología Del Deporte 21(2):183–197

Oliveira R, Brito JP, Moreno-Villanueva A, Nalha M, Rico-González M, Clemente FM (2021c) Reference values for external and internal training intensity monitoring in young male soccer players: a systematic review. Healthcare (Switzerland) 9(11):1–16. https://doi.org/10.3390/healthcare9111567

Oliveira R, Martins AD, Moreno-Villanueva A, Brito JP, Nalha M, Rico-González M, Clemente FM (2022) Reference values for external and internal load training intensity monitoring in professional male soccer players: a systematic review. Int J Sports Sci Coach 17:1506. https://doi.org/10.1177/17479541211072966

Plisk S, Stone M (2003) Periodization strategies. Strength Cond J 25(6):19. https://doi.org/10.1519/1533-4295

Rico-González M, Mendez-Villanueva A, Los Arcos A (2020) Training load periodization in soccer with one official match a week: a systematic review. In: Raya-González J, Mendez-Villanueva A, Arcos AL (eds) An essential guide to sports performance. Nova science

Staunton CA, Abt G, Weaving D, Wundersitz DWT (2021) Misuse of the term 'load' in sport and exercise science. J Sci Med Sport 25:439. https://doi.org/10.1016/j.jsams.2021.08.013

Stevens T, Ruiter C, Twisk L, Savelsbergh G, Beek P (2017) Quantification of in-season training load relative to match load in professional Dutch Eredivisie football players. Sci Med Footb 1(2):117–125. https://doi.org/10.1080/24733938.2017.1282163

Thorpe RT, Strudwick AJ, Buchheit M, Atkinson G, Drust B, Gregson W (2016) Tracking morning fatigue status across in-season training weeks in elite soccer players. Int J Sports Physiol Perform 11:947–952. https://doi.org/10.1123/ijspp.2015-0490

Weston M (2018) Training load monitoring in elite English soccer: a comparison of practices and perceptions between coaches and practitioners. Sci Med Footb 2(3):216–224. https://doi.org/10.1080/24733938.2018.1427883

Building a Monitoring System

9

Paweł Chmura, Marek Konefał, Marcin Andrzejewski,
and Arne Jaspers

The application of an appropriate monitoring strategy enables subsequent adjustments to be made more effective in the training process to ensure that the program continues the desired outcomes. Without such monitoring strategy, any decision-making becomes dependent on subjective opinions largely based on experience and will lack the foundation of objective information. The combination of objective information and subjective experiences can contribute to a successful coaching process. Currently, an array of tools is available to support the assessment of training load. Practitioners and sports scientists should continually evaluate the multiple data streams in contributing to the global aims of conditioning in professional soccer, such as maintaining and/or enhancing various fitness attributes, optimizing readiness for competition, and keeping players' injury risk low. There are some clear benefits in the accurate understanding of the training load for individual players. This understanding ensures that the performance is not compromised by exposing players to too little or too much load and provide the ability to evaluate if training demands are appropriate when compared to known match demands. They also enable the evaluation of a specific session or drill to see if the desired loads are achieved and allow players to be monitored during rehabilitation to ensure that an appropriate return to training takes place.

P. Chmura (✉)
Department of Team Games, University School of Physical Education, Wrocław, Poland

M. Konefał
Department of Biological and Motor Sport Bases, University School of Physical Education, Wrocław, Poland

M. Andrzejewski
Department of Methodology of Recreation, Poznań University of Physical Education, Poznań, Poland

A. Jaspers
KU Leuven, Faculty of Movement and Rehabilitation Sciences, Leuven, Belgium

J. M. Oliva Lozano, L. P. Ardigò (eds.), *Training Load in Professional Soccer*,
https://doi.org/10.1007/978-3-031-52087-7_9

9.1 Introduction

Currently, professional soccer players play about 50–60 matches (and even more) per season including domestic league, continental tournaments, national cups, and national team matches (Chmura et al. 2019). The global burden of injuries consists of an average of 2.0 injuries per player per season and an injury incidence of 8.0 injuries per 1000 h of training and match exposure (Ekstrand et al. 2011). Therefore, the availability of players for training and matches is a main goal for the coaching staff. Various research studies showed that player availability is an important factor for success in professional team sports, which highlights the importance of systematic monitoring of training load, and the use of injury prevention strategies (Ekstrand et al. 2021; Hägglund et al. 2013). Given the physical and mental load placed upon the modern player, training programs that prepare a player for competition while reducing his or her susceptibility to extensive fatigue, injury, and illness are fundamental to the work of the athlete's support of the team (Gregson et al. 2018).

Load management has become a critical area of current sports science practices. It is commonly employed to improve and/or maintain physical performance and accelerate recovery while reducing susceptibility to extensive fatigue, injury, and illness (Rago 2019). Indeed, players have become more familiar with regular assessments, wearable training load (TL) monitoring technology incorporating global navigation satellite systems (GNSS), or heart rate (HR) monitors (Coutts et al. 2018), as well as self-reported questionnaires (e.g., post-session rating of perceived exertion [RPE]). These technological advances are considered an added value for decision-making regarding the training process (Houtmeyers et al. 2021). Inappropriate training progressions can be identified and inform coaches on suitable alternatives (Brink and Frencken 2018). However, the abundance of player monitoring tools may cause confusion about the training dose-player response to which different data are expected to be associated (Rago 2019; Vanrenterghem et al. 2017).

9.2 The General Guidelines of Good Monitoring Practices

From a practical perspective, the benefits of monitoring for athletes need to be clarified. They should consist of an individualized design of training routines to enhance performance and well-being (Gabbett et al. 2017). In coordination with the athletic staff, suitable monitoring instruments should be selected based on previously specified goals. This decision also depends on aspects such as schedule, availability of time, financial resources, or other organizational considerations. For example, monitoring at defined key moments (preseason, in-season, and postseason) or selected intervals (preseason—first competition) during a season could be conducted with more effort and investment in terms of financial and staff resources (Heidari et al. 2019). Educated and experienced staff could engage to obtain multidimensional reference values for the recovery status. This mode of operation is indicated for the analysis of long-term developments or the comprehensive analysis of training camps or longer-lasting competitions. Ideally, a combination of key assessments at certain points and regular monitoring (e.g., weekly, monthly) with brief measures (e.g., Multicomponent Training Distress Scale [MTDS]) is recommended (Saw et al. 2016). This approach helps to develop targeted interventions for monitored athletes. With the extensive information gathered from assessments at the important time points, long-term interventions can be designed. By contrast, regular monitoring with shorter instruments may serve as an immediate indicator of the recovery status, resulting in acute interventions (Heidari et al. 2019).

With the appropriate manipulation of data and efficient data management systems, practitioners can be informed quickly of key monitoring variables: new loads, changes in load, chronic loads, and acute versus chronic loads or training stress balance. These all have implications for how players are subsequently managed to reduce injury risk and optimize performance. Whether insights are being made from session reports or weekly reports, similar questions are being asked, ultimately guiding practice to elicit optimal responses to enhance players' abilities while maximizing their readiness for competition. A general premise is that there is a holistic plan to the training week while within the week players are micromanaged accordingly. The monitoring of training load and recovery is integral to the delivery of a suitable training plan (Bourdon et al. 2017). If accurate and easy-to-interpret feedback is provided to the athlete and coach, load monitoring can result in enhanced knowledge of training responses, aid in the design of training programs, provide a further avenue for communication between support staff and athletes and coaches, and ultimately enhance an athlete's performance (Halson 2014).

Despite the numerous studies and reviews on monitoring, no gold standard monitoring structure for teams has been identified (Bourdon et al. 2017; Lambert and Borresen 2010). An explanation for this is that frequent monitoring of athletes is not easily managed due to the often-limited resources and time required to conduct a monitoring session. In team sports, there are diverse training activities within the team, yet the players have to be managed simultaneously. This adds an extra logistical challenge to monitoring (Starling and Lambert 2018).

9.3 Challenges When Building a Monitoring Strategy

One of the challenges sports scientists, analysts, and physical preparation trainers face is that, during a training process, huge amounts of data can be monitored on a daily/weekly basis. Vanrenterghem et al. (2017) indicated that turning this data into relevant information for players, coaches, and therapists can be an extremely daunting challenge. It is apparent that the potential exists to collect a vast amount of information from which to make suitable assessments of training load. It is important, however, that data are not collected merely for the sake of it and that the potential "data tsunami" is managed appropriately; the information obtained via the chosen methods needs to be used to impact upon the coaching process (Gregson et al. 2018).

The practical implementation of athlete monitoring systems poses a particular challenge due to the complex and multidimensional structure of game demands and player and team performance. Ideally, a comprehensive monitoring system includes markers for all relevant biopsychosociological aspects of training and performance, combining them into a holistic approach (Heidari et al. 2019). Another great challenge is, therefore, the implementation of a simple but effective monitoring system that involves at least some measures of training load, wellness, fitness, and readiness (Gabbett et al. 2017; McGuigan 2017). The frequent assessment of various metrics could be difficult as compliance can be affected by the busy schedule and complex requirements of the team sport athlete (Schneider et al. 2018).

An adequate use of scientific and statistical methods can improve the confidence of decisions made from athlete monitoring data (Thornton et al. 2019). In team sports, sport scientists and support staff often collect a wide range of athlete monitoring data. They relate to external and internal training loads that their athletes have undergone, as well as physiological and psychological assessments of fatigue (Halson 2014). When appropriately collected and interpreted, these data should inform decision-making processes regarding the planning and manipulation of training (Thornton et al. 2019). While it is essential for athlete monitoring systems to have strong proof of concept for its design and consist of valid and reliable measures, the effectiveness of the system is dependent on how well the data can be used to inform coaching and training decisions. In high-performance sport, decisions around manipulating training need to be relayed to the coach within a brief period prior to training commencing. Traditionally, a heavy reliance has been placed upon identifying trends in monitoring data visually (Coutts et al. 2018). Therefore, recent research suggests the application of comprehensible and transparent statistics, such as graphs and the visualization of the smallest meaningful change (Batterham and Hopkins 2006), which can then be communicated directly to the athletes and coaches (Buchheit 2017; Gabbett et al. 2017). For example, a simple reporting method used to demonstrate a change in monitoring variables is through a traffic light alert system to identify "red flags" (Heidari et al. 2019; Robertson et al. 2017). The systematically collected data should be synthesized according to the knowledge and background of the target population of athletes. As a final and essential outcome of monitoring, training routines in team or individual contexts can be adapted and individualized recovery strategies can be implemented (Kellmann et al. 2018).

Williams et al. (2017) stated that the challenge from a practitioner's perspective is to decide which measures they should calculate and monitor in their athletes. With respect to analyzing the association between training load measures and injury risk or performance, many of the variables are likely to be highly correlated with one another, and so including several of these measures within an analysis may not be advisable for statistical reasons (i.e., multicollinearity) (Hair et al. 2010). The reduction of these factors to the most parsimonious set of variables, which still convey the underlying dimensions of the data, would be desirable for practitioners. Ryan et al. (2021) highlighted that one approach to address the issue of data overload in athlete monitoring is to selectively reduce the number of variables that are collected and analyzed to improve the efficiency of analysis without losing the veracity of the information provided by these data. One such method is principal component analysis (PCA), a data reduction technique designed to evaluate the contribution of multiple variables to the variance of an entire dataset of correlated measures (Ryan et al. 2021; Weaving et al. 2018; Williams et al. 2017). This method selects the key performance indicators and disregards the least important components of the analysis (Oliva-Lozano et al. 2021a, b; Parmar et al. 2018). More advanced analysis methods, such as machine learning (Rossi et al. 2018), do not have to be considered as the holy grail, but could provide additional insights in the relation between multiple load and response indicators. Jaspers et al. (2018) indicated that the advantage of using the data-driven approach of machine learning is the ability to detect possible interplayer differences.

9.4 Monitoring the Training Process

Exercise acts as a stressor, triggering a range of psychophysiological responses that, in turn, facilitate cellular adaptations across multiple organ systems (Impellizzeri et al. 2019). To obtain optimal training adaptations, a careful balance between training dose and recovery is required (Matveyev 1981) and to achieve specific performance adaptations, training should focus on the systems that play a crucial role in determining performance (Impellizzeri et al. 2019). Thus, once acute fatigue has dissipated, improved performance is expected after a given period (Coutts et al. 2018). The training process describes the systematic and periodized application of physiological and biomechanical stress in pursuit of functional training outcomes (Impellizzeri et al. 2005). The development or maintenance of fitness and the potentiation of biomotor abilities are two outcomes that are important to prepare intermittent team sport athletes for the frequent and substantial demands of competition (Iaia et al. 2009). Such adaptations are determined by a combination of training volume, intensity, and frequency (Coffey and Hawley 2007), collectively referred to as training load (Banister et al. 1975; Foster et al. 2001; Kenttä and Hassmén 1998; McLaren et al. 2018). Training load is the input variable in a training system that coaches and scientists most commonly manipulate to elicit the desired training response. As such, quantifying and monitoring training load should form the foundation of any athlete monitoring system (Coutts et al. 2018). Training load encompasses both external and internal dimensions, with external training loads representing the physical work performed during the training session or match and internal training loads being the associated biochemical (physical and physiological) and biomechanical stress responses (Vanrenterghem et al. 2017).

The recent development of sophisticated (micro)technology now allows for increasingly detailed information about external load considered recently as "gold standard" or "criterion measures" (Cardinale and Varley 2017). For example, with the use of GNSS, accelerometers, and gyroscopes, it is now relatively simple to quantify accelerations, decelerations, speed, and power during exercise (Impellizzeri et al. 2019). In team sports, the external load can be described by measures such as distance covered in specific speed zones, accelerations, or metabolic power (it infers metabolism, which is internal to the athlete); the latter is mathematically derived from the speed–time profile and therefore remains an external load indicator

(Gregson et al. 2018). Recently, Morin et al. (2021) examined one of the most promising concepts of speed monitoring. They presented a method to derive the players' individual acceleration–speed (AS) profile in situ, i.e., from global positioning system data collected over several soccer sessions (without running specific tests). For more details on external load measures, see Chap. 3.

The internal load, or the relative physiological and psychological strain resulting from the external training factors, is crucial in determining both the stress imposed and the subsequent adaptation to training (Halson 2014). This type of load is considered the ultimate stimulus for training adaptations (Viru and Viru 2000) and results from the interaction between the external load and the individual or intrinsic characteristics of a player (Bouchard and Rankinen 2001; Jaspers et al. 2017). Resting HR, HR response to exercise (HRex), and HR recovery (HRR) following exercise are simple measures that can be collected from athletes in the training setting—and have been reported to have some utility for assessing athlete fitness (Coutts et al. 2018). Another simple and time-efficient method to evaluate internal load is the session-RPE, as a global rating of session intensity (Foster et al. 2001). Questionnaires and diaries can be also a relatively simple and inexpensive means of determining the training load and subsequent responses to that training. Biochemical monitoring is also an important part of internal load monitoring. For more details on internal load measures, see Chap. 3.

Sport scientists, practitioners, and coaches are constantly looking for new solutions on how to develop multidimensional monitoring systems. It is considered that an integrated approach, rigorous and consistent, combining the use of internal and external loads, provides more significant information about the stress caused in soccer players than interpretations based on isolated data (Bourdon et al. 2017; Jaspers et al. 2017; Miguel et al. 2021). Several studies have identified the importance of contextualizing physiological and perceptual measures with training load, particularly during intensified training periods (Aubry et al. 2015; Bellenger et al. 2016). The integrated physiological assessment of both training outcome and process allows researchers (1) to improve interpretation of physical tests used to verify the effectiveness of training programs, (2) to evaluate the organization of the training load in order to design periodization strategies, (3) to identify athletes who are poor responders, (4) to control the compliance of the training completed to that planned by the coach, and (5) to modify the training process before the assessment of its outcome, thus optimizing soccer performance (Impellizzeri et al. 2005).

Whereas this model appears simple to understand, soccer literature showed that this is not always the case. A higher training dose over time seems to be beneficial for isokinetic strength, trivial for body composition, whereas controversial results (either beneficial or harmful) have been reported for sprint, jump aerobic, and anaerobic fitness (Jaspers et al. 2017). Therefore, the dose–response relationship between TL and training outcome requires further investigations. External load can be easily quantified during analytic exercises, once exercise duration, running distance, and recovery time between bouts are known, even though the internal load can vary between and within individuals. Nonetheless, quantifying external training load during skill- or game-based exercises can be challenging, with variations in locomotor, physiological, and perceptual responses observed according to different external factors, such as pitch dimension, number of players, exercise regime, game rules, etc. (Hill-Haas et al. 2011; Rago 2019). The monitoring of training load is therefore an important aspect of athlete management (Bourdon et al. 2017; Schwellnus et al. 2016; Soligard et al. 2016) and has the potential to provide practitioners and coaches with an objective framework for evidence-based decisions (Gabbett et al. 2016; McLaren et al. 2018).

Newton et al. (2019) indicated that practitioners are able to measure the physiological stress the players are exposed to by the prescribed training (Fig. 9.1).

Because of advances in technology over the past decade, numerous concepts, frameworks, and monitoring methods are available to coaches and sports scientists to evaluate the various training and match load components. They all have their advantages and disadvantages. The concept that is adopted generally depends on the training culture, coaching philosophy, and budget. While each of these measures helps to understand the training process for athletes, the value of load monitoring is increased when these measures are contextualized against each other and also against the athlete's fitness and fatigue responses to training (Coutts et al. 2018). Regardless of which methods are adopted, the validity and reliability of the data remain crucial, and it should also be acknowledged that the power of the information increases over time since a longitudinal profile enables far more detailed analysis to be carried out to support the decision-making processes that ultimately enable players to perform to their potential (Gregson et al. 2018).

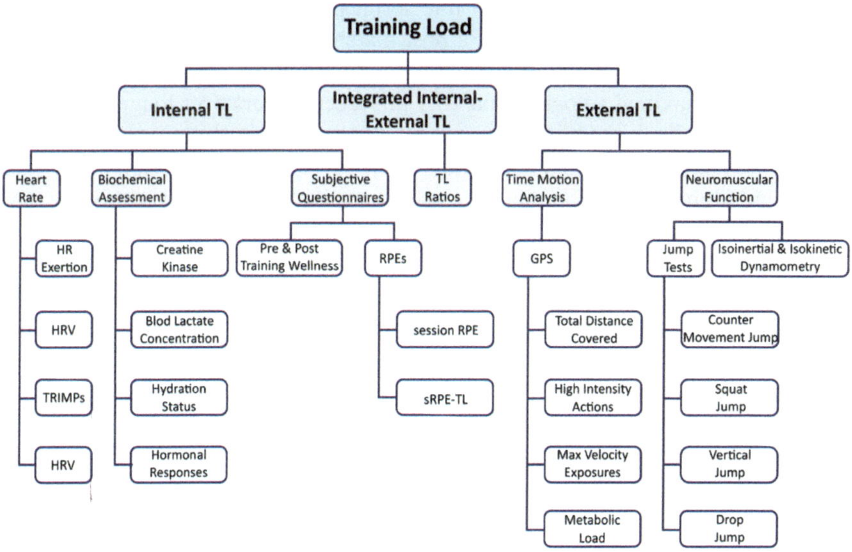

Fig. 9.1 Training load measures presented by Newton et al. (2019). *TL* training load, *HRV* heart rate variability, *TRIMP* training impulse, *RPE* rating of perceived exertion, *GPS* global positioning systems. (Reproduced from Newton et al. (2019) under the terms and conditions of the Creative Commons Attribution (CC BY) 4.0 International License)

9.5 Application of Exercise Tests

Adjusting optimal and individualized training loads requires frequent monitoring of changes in physical qualities (Buchheit 2014). Without regular fitness measures, it is difficult to accurately determine if athletes are adapting to training, and/or if the athlete's fitness status has been adequately developed. Anecdotally, it is often questioned after poor performance if the result was due to lack of fitness or other physical capacities. It needs to be highlighted that conducting maximal performance tests for physical qualities of elite soccer players, especially during in-season phases, is challenged by poor player compliance, time constraints because of congested match schedules (Carling et al. 2015), and practitioners' perceived increased risk of injury (McCall et al. 2014; Rabbani et al. 2020). Criteria for a fitness test that can be included into a monitoring system should be that it is valid, reliable, be able to accurately reflect training status, be cost-effective, and easy to implement with minimal disruption to normal training. Accordingly, recent focus has aimed to develop non-fatigue-inducing fitness tests that assess physiological responses (i.e., HR, blood lactate, and RPE) to standardized submaximal work (Buchheit 2014; Buchheit et al. 2012, 2013; Crowcroft et al. 2015). This research has resulted in the development of simple field tests assessing HR responses to standard bouts of exercise to monitor athletes' acute and chronic fitness adaptations to training (Buchheit 2014; Coutts et al. 2018).

As soccer is a sport mainly involving horizontal motions, sprint testing might be a more appropriate means for evaluating real-world performance rather than jump assessments. However, short straight-line sprint performance (e.g., 10–20 m) has recently shown to lack sensitivity as a post-match (24–48 h) indicator of physical fatigue in semiprofessional soccer players (Brownstein et al. 2017). Analysis of decrements in maximal velocity capability in soccer players over longer sprint distances (30 m) is suggested to improve evaluation of fatigue following match play (Nagahara et al. 2016). Again, constraints related to sprint testing (e.g., injury risk, additional fatigue, player compliance, coach "buy-in," place of test within the day-to-day working practices) need to be carefully evaluated. Carling et al. (2018) critically assessed the use of tests during the season. Similarly, assessments such as a countermovement jump (CMJ) on a portable platform are quick and easy means of determining neuromuscular fatigue. Yet, in applied settings, there can be reluctance by coaches, support staff, and players themselves to perform such tests as they are explosive in nature and require maximal effort and additional loading. These factors reduce the applicability even when testing is performed conveniently following a customary warm-up prior to training. Motivating individuals not to perform assessments is also essential but not easy in practice, while practitioners must ensure players do not alter mechanics in an attempt to maximize jump performance (Taylor et al. 2012). Finally, consensus is necessary on the choice of variables measured during jump testing. For example, the ratio of flight time to contraction time is shown to be a more sensitive measure of recovery compared to jump height in professional soccer players performing a CMJ (Carling et al. 2018; Rowell et al. 2017).

9.6 Data Analysis

Lacome et al. (2018) presented a practical framework for applying statistics in the field of sport science. Essentially, the process of data analysis should commence by evaluating the typical error of measurement (TE) for each metric (or obtain it from existing literature) and calculating the smallest worthwhile change (SWC). Once these variables are defined, the framework employs magnitude-based inferences to compare the change or difference in the variable of interest (±TE) with the SWC. Consequently, this approach provides the staff with meaningful results that the likelihood of change can be assessed.

With the development of integrated monitoring systems, there is a need for stronger evidence to highlight the likelihood of a particular outcome (i.e., injury, illness, or change in performance) (Taylor et al. 2012). Coutts et al. (2018) indicated that a multidimensional monitoring system could be required to improve the diagnostic accuracy of athlete monitoring systems. A common analytical approach used to assess if monitoring variables are effective to identify an outcome is to compare the accuracy of a monitoring cutoff value against a binary outcome (e.g., Did performance improve?—yes or no). These values can then be applied to quantify the accuracy and optimal cutoff values to inform decision-makers of the likelihood of an outcome (Fawcett 2006). Furthermore, when interpreting changes in such responses, individualized methods may be used, such as Z-scores, to highlight the relative change in the variable. Means and standard deviations (SD) should be reported, as these depict the variation in the responses, reflecting the effect of the treatment between individuals. The SD at baseline may be used to assess the magnitudes of effects and individual responses by standardization (Hopkins 2015). These data may be reported at the individual or group level, where the mean and SD of the change scores for each experimental group is depicted (Hopkins 2015). Additionally, confidence intervals (CIs) may be included, as CIs are effective in providing the true value of the variance of individual responses (Batterham and Hopkins 2006; Thornton et al. 2019).

9.7 Effective Feedback

Player feedback and indirect estimates of work volume are useful monitoring tools. However, systematic laboratory and/or field-based performance tests (Kannas et al. 2015; Krustrup et al. 2003; López-Segovia et al. 2014), quantification of GPS/accelerometer monitoring (Dwyer and Gabbett 2012; Scott et al. 2013; Wehbe et al. 2014), and training volume via heart rate monitoring (Kalapotharakos et al. 2011) enable strength and conditioning coaches and players to make more informed, data-driven training decisions (Huggins et al. 2019). The first step to build a monitoring system is to ensure that a measurement tool is valid and reliable. Then, decisions around athletes may be based on small fluctuations, and thus, precision is extremely important to differentiate between real change and measurement error. Taken together, these assumptions can add scientific legitimacy and meaningfulness to the data expression to athletes and coaches (Halson 2014; Robertson et al. 2017). Data from fitness tests provide an insight into players' capacity and together with TL quantification can objectively inform about the training process. Despite external training load being the main determinant of internal training load, other factors such as genetic, training background, and starting fitness level could influence the exercise response imposed on the individual and, ultimately, the training outcome (Impellizzeri et al. 2005). Indeed, athletes repeating the same exercise on different moments over time may maintain the same exercise output but experience different physiological and perceptual responses (Rago 2019).

Thornton et al. (2019) provided a methodological outline that may assist team sport practitioners to develop and employ simple and effective feedback for coaches and athletes. The following steps may be considered (Thornton et al. 2019):

Step 1. Considerations for player monitoring in team sports:

- Clearly define the objectives of the athlete monitoring system. Specify what aspects you aim to measure or evaluate, such as fitness levels, fatigue, injury, or illness risks.
- Understand the needs of key stakeholders, including coaches and athletes.
- Acknowledge logistical and financial constraints.
- Identify variables that are both valid and reliable for measuring the desired outcomes. Focus on variables that capture fitness, fatigue, and potential risks related to injury or illness.

Step 2. Methods of analyzing data:

- Determine where the collected data will be stored and analyze, considering options such as commercial athlete monitoring systems or tools like Microsoft Excel.
- Assess whether additional analyses, such as acute:chronic workload ratio, z scores, or standard tens scores, are needed based on the data type and the goals of the monitoring system.

Step 3. Determining meaningful changes in data:

- Decide on a method to evaluate meaningful changes in data. Options include typical error, effect sizes, coefficient of variation, or smallest worthwhile change.
- Select a method that is quick and efficient for timely decision-making.

Step 4. Establish effective methods to present and communicate important information:

- Select the most relevant information to present (e.g., key parameters).
- Choose appropriate data visualization/presentation tools.
- Ensure that the information is conveyed in a clear and understandable manner, facilitating informed decision-making.

Düking et al. (2018) also presented an integrated framework of load monitoring by a combination of smartphone applications, wearables, and point-of-care testing

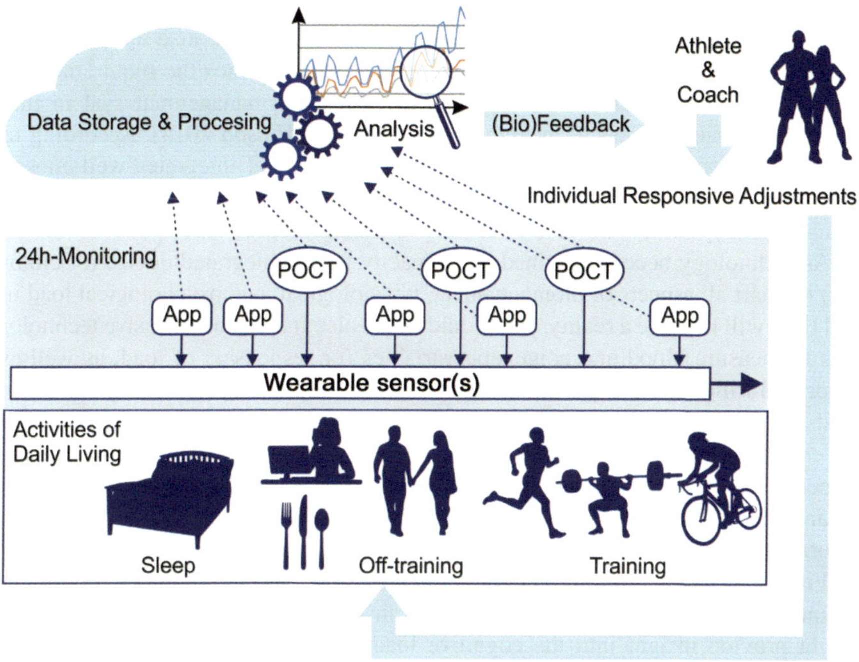

Fig. 9.2 Procedure for monitoring external and internal training load-employing apps, wearables, and point-of-care testing (POCT) and providing feedback to athletes and their coaches that allows beneficial responsive modification of exercise programs (Düking et al. 2018). (Reproduced from Düking et al. 2018, under the terms and conditions of the Creative Commons Attribution (CC BY) license (http://creativecommons.org/licenses/by/4.0/))

that provides feedback that allows individual responsive adjustments to activities of daily living. The framework presented by him clearly shows the trend of an increasingly broader approach to collecting data about individual players or teams. Systemically, more information is collected not only from before, during, and after training, but also in the periods between training. The aim is to monitor the condition of the body and the response to effort around the clock, week, or month, in order to have the best possible insight into what is happening with the athlete's body. Figure 9.2 illustrates a procedure for individualized management of load and recovery designed to optimize performance and/or minimize the risk of overuse, injury, and/or illnesses.

9.8 Perspectives and Future Directions

With the rate of development in miniature technology, wearable analytic tools, and apps, it is relatively easy to predict that the sport scientist, athlete, and coach of the future will have access to more sensing solutions for predicting and coordinating performance than ever before (Bourdon et al. 2017). Furthermore, with the increasing amounts of data available from monitoring devices such as GPS, digital video, photocells and ergometers, in combination with internal load measurements such as HR, questionnaires, and perceptions of fatigue comes the requirement to incorporate this information into a database and data management system that results in efficient access to meaningful information (Halson 2014). According to Pyne and Martin (2011), "a systems-based approach that integrates well-chosen diagnostic tests, with smart sensor technology and a real-time database and data management system, is the future for fatigue management in elite sport."

As technology becomes refined, the capacity for an integrated device (or clothing) to chart all aspects of biomechanical, physiological, and psychological load in real time will become a reality. This could likely also include noninvasive technologies to measure blood and epigenetic variables (or responses) of load, as well as report calorific intake/expenditure and recovery processes (sleep, etc.) (Bourdon et al. 2017). The challenge will be to ensure that the programmers can understand the context of the data (for each given sport/event) and that data can be presented in a meaningful manner to athletes and coaches. The ability to visualize data in a meaningful way will be crucial to ensure that training load activities are able to inform and influence the coaching process.

Finally, fatigued athletes often report impaired concentration and cognitive complaints (McMorris et al. 2018). Therefore, investigation into psychomotor speed might provide insight into the cognitive load induced by exercise (Chmura and Nazar 2010). Future research may include developing concepts, methods, and training measures to help athletes break the fatigue barrier (at the brain level) (Davranche and McMorris 2009). So that by tolerating higher and higher intensity during training and a match for longer and longer periods of time, they maintain high efficiency of actions and the speed of making the right decisions. It will also be extremely important in the future to develop tools to monitor the fastest possible regeneration and return of the player to the pitch (Thorpe et al. 2015).

References

Aubry A, Hausswirth C, Louis J, Coutts AJ, Buchheit M, le Meur Y (2015) The development of functional overreaching is associated with a faster heart rate recovery in endurance athletes. PLoS One 10(10):e0139754. https://doi.org/10.1371/journal.pone.0139754

Banister EW, Calvert TW, Savage MV, Bach T (1975) A systems model of training for athletic performance. Aust J Sports Med Exerc Sci 7:57–61

Batterham AM, Hopkins WG (2006) Making meaningful inferences about magnitudes. Int J Sports Physiol Perform 1(1):50–57. https://doi.org/10.1123/ijspp.1.1.50

Bellenger CR, Karavirta L, Thomson RL, Robertson EY, Davison K, Buckley JD (2016) Contextualizing parasympathetic hyperactivity in functionally overreached athletes with perceptions of training tolerance. Int J Sports Physiol Perform 11(5):685–692. https://doi.org/10.1123/ijspp.2015-0495

Bouchard C, Rankinen T (2001) Individual differences in response to regular physical activity. Med Sci Sports Exerc 33(Supplement):S446–S451. https://doi.org/10.1097/00005768-200106001-00013

Bourdon PC, Cardinale M, Murray A, Gastin P, Kellmann M, Varley MC, Gabbett TJ, Coutts AJ, Burgess DJ, Gregson W, Cable NT (2017) Monitoring athlete training loads: consensus

statement. Int J Sports Physiol Perform 12(Suppl 2):S2161–S2170. https://doi.org/10.1123/IJSPP.2017-0208
Brink MS, Frencken WGP (2018) Formative feedback for the coach reduces mismatch between coach and players' perceptions of exertion. Sci Med Footb 2(4):255–260. https://doi.org/10.1080/24733938.2018.1451651
Brownstein CG, Dent JP, Parker P, Hicks KM, Howatson G, Goodall S, Thomas K (2017) Etiology and recovery of neuromuscular fatigue following competitive soccer match-play. Front Physiol 8:831. https://doi.org/10.3389/fphys.2017.00831
Buchheit M (2014) Monitoring training status with HR measures: do all roads lead to Rome? Front Physiol 5:73. https://doi.org/10.3389/fphys.2014.00073
Buchheit M (2017) Houston, we still have a problem. Int J Sports Physiol Perform 12(8):1111–1114. https://doi.org/10.1123/ijspp.2017-0422
Buchheit M, Simpson MB, al Haddad H, Bourdon PC, Mendez-Villanueva A (2012) Monitoring changes in physical performance with heart rate measures in young soccer players. Eur J Appl Physiol 112(2):711–723. https://doi.org/10.1007/s00421-011-2014-0
Buchheit M, Racinais S, Bilsborough JC, Bourdon PC, Voss SC, Hocking J, Cordy J, Mendez-Villanueva A, Coutts AJ (2013) Monitoring fitness, fatigue and running performance during a pre-season training camp in elite football players. J Sci Med Sport 16(6):550–555. https://doi.org/10.1016/j.jsams.2012.12.003
Cardinale M, Varley MC (2017) Wearable training-monitoring technology: applications, challenges, and opportunities. Int J Sports Physiol Perform 12(s2):S2-55-S2-62. https://doi.org/10.1123/ijspp.2016-0423
Carling C, Gregson W, McCall A, Moreira A, Wong DP, Bradley PS (2015) Match running performance during fixture congestion in elite soccer: research issues and future directions. Sports Med 45(5):605–613. https://doi.org/10.1007/s40279-015-0313-z
Carling C, Lacome M, McCall A, Dupont G, le Gall F, Simpson B, Buchheit M (2018) Monitoring of post-match fatigue in professional soccer: welcome to the real world. Sports Med 48(12):2695–2702. https://doi.org/10.1007/s40279-018-0935-z
Chmura J, Nazar K (2010) Parallel changes in the onset of blood lactate accumulation (OBLA) and threshold of psychomotor performance deterioration during incremental exercise after training in athletes. Int J Psychophysiol 75(3):287–290. https://doi.org/10.1016/j.ijpsycho.2009.12.011
Chmura P, Konefał M, Wong DP, Figueiredo AJ, Kowalczuk E, Rokita A, Chmura J, Andrzejewski M (2019) Players' physical performance decreased after two-thirds of the season: results of 3 consecutive seasons in the German first Bundesliga. Int J Environ Res Public Health 16(11):2044. https://doi.org/10.3390/ijerph16112044
Coffey VG, Hawley JA (2007) The molecular bases of training adaptation. Sports Med 37(9):737–763. https://doi.org/10.2165/00007256-200737090-00001
Coutts AJ, Crowcroft S, Kempton T (2018) Developing athlete monitoring systems: theoretical basis and practical applications. In: Kellmann M, Beckmann J (eds) Sport, recovery and performance: interdisciplinary insights. Routledge, pp 19–32
Crowcroft S, Duffield R, McCleave E, Slattery K, Wallace LK, Coutts AJ (2015) Monitoring training to assess changes in fitness and fatigue: the effects of training in heat and hypoxia. Scand J Med Sci Sports 25:287–295. https://doi.org/10.1111/sms.12364
Davranche K, McMorris T (2009) Specific effects of acute moderate exercise on cognitive control. Brain Cogn 69(3):565–570. https://doi.org/10.1016/j.bandc.2008.12.001
Düking P, Achtzehn S, Holmberg H-C, Sperlich B (2018) Integrated framework of load monitoring by a combination of smartphone applications, wearables and point-of-care testing provides feedback that allows individual responsive adjustments to activities of daily living. Sensors 18(5):1632. https://doi.org/10.3390/s18051632
Dwyer DB, Gabbett TJ (2012) Global positioning system data analysis: velocity ranges and a new definition of sprinting for field sport athletes. J Strength Cond Res 26(3):818–824. https://doi.org/10.1519/JSC.0b013e3182276555
Ekstrand J, Hagglund M, Walden M (2011) Injury incidence and injury patterns in professional football: the UEFA injury study. Br J Sports Med 45(7):553–558. https://doi.org/10.1136/bjsm.2009.060582

Ekstrand J, Spreco A, Bengtsson H, Bahr R (2021) Injury rates decreased in men's professional football: an 18-year prospective cohort study of almost 12 000 injuries sustained during 1.8 million hours of play. Br J Sports Med 55(19):1084–1092. https://doi.org/10.1136/bjsports-2020-103159

Fawcett T (2006) An introduction to ROC analysis. Pattern Recogn Lett 27(8):861–874. https://doi.org/10.1016/j.patrec.2005.10.010

Foster C, Florhaug JA, Franklin J, Gottschall L, Hrovatin LA, Parker S, Doleshal P, Dodge C (2001) A new approach to monitoring exercise training. J Strength Cond Res 15(1):109–115

Gabbett HT, Windt J, Gabbett TJ (2016) Cost-benefit analysis underlies training decisions in elite sport. Br J Sports Med 50(21):1291–1292. https://doi.org/10.1136/bjsports-2016-096079

Gabbett TJ, Nassis GP, Oetter E, Pretorius J, Johnston N, Medina D, Rodas G, Myslinski T, Howells D, Beard A, Ryan A (2017) The athlete monitoring cycle: a practical guide to interpreting and applying training monitoring data. Br J Sports Med 51(20):1451–1452. https://doi.org/10.1136/bjsports-2016-097298

Gregson W, Hawkins R, Thorpe RT (2018) Monitoring player load and fatigue status. In: Gregson W, Littlewood M (eds) Science in soccer: translating theory into practice, 1st edn. Bloomsbury Sport Publishing, pp 122–149

Hägglund M, Waldén M, Magnusson H, Kristenson K, Bengtsson H, Ekstrand J (2013) Injuries affect team performance negatively in professional football: an 11-year follow-up of the UEFA champions league injury study. Br J Sports Med 47(12):738–742. https://doi.org/10.1136/bjsports-2013-092215

Hair JF Jr, Anderson RE, Babin BJ, Black WC (2010) Multivariate data analysis: a global perspective, 7th edn. Pearson education, Upper Saddle River, NJ; http://lib.ugent.be/catalog/rug01:001321386

Halson SL (2014) Monitoring training load to understand fatigue in athletes. Sports Med 44(S2):139–147. https://doi.org/10.1007/s40279-014-0253-z

Heidari J, Beckmann J, Bertollo M, Brink M, Kallus KW, Robazza C, Kellmann M (2019) Multidimensional monitoring of recovery status and implications for performance. Int J Sports Physiol Perform 14(1):2–8. https://doi.org/10.1123/ijspp.2017-0669

Hill-Haas SV, Dawson B, Impellizzeri FM, Coutts AJ (2011) Physiology of small-sided games training in football. Sports Med 41(3):199–220. https://doi.org/10.2165/11539740-000000000-00000

Hopkins WG (2015) Individual responses made easy. J Appl Physiol 118(12):1444–1446. https://doi.org/10.1152/japplphysiol.00098.2015

Houtmeyers KC, Jaspers A, Figueiredo P (2021) Managing the Training Process in Elite Sports: From Descriptive to Prescriptive Data Analytics. Int J Sports Physiol Perform 16(11):1719–1723. https://doi.org/10.1123/ijspp.2020-0958

Huggins RA, Fortunati AR, Curtis RM, Looney DP, West CA, Lee EC, Fragala MS, Hall ML, Casa DJ (2019) Monitoring blood biomarkers and training load throughout a collegiate soccer season. J Strength Cond Res 33(11):3065–3077. https://doi.org/10.1519/JSC.0000000000002622

Iaia FM, Ermanno R, Bangsbo J (2009) High-intensity training in football. Int J Sports Physiol Perform 4(3):291–306. https://doi.org/10.1123/ijspp.4.3.291

Impellizzeri FM, Rampinini E, Marcora SM (2005) Physiological assessment of aerobic training in soccer. J Sports Sci 23(6):583–592. https://doi.org/10.1080/02640410400021278

Impellizzeri FM, Marcora SM, Coutts AJ (2019) Internal and external training load: 15 years on. Int J Sports Physiol Perform 14(2):270–273. https://doi.org/10.1123/ijspp.2018-0935

Jaspers A, Brink MS, Probst SGM, Frencken WGP, Helsen WF (2017) Relationships between training load indicators and training outcomes in professional soccer. Sports Med 47(3):533–544. https://doi.org/10.1007/s40279-016-0591-0

Jaspers A, de Beéck TO, Brink MS, Frencken WGP, Staes F, Davis JJ, Helsen WF (2018) Relationships between the external and internal training load in professional soccer: what can we learn from machine learning? Int J Sports Physiol Perform 13(5):625–630. https://doi.org/10.1123/ijspp.2017-0299

Kalapotharakos VI, Ziogas G, Tokmakidis SP (2011) Seasonal aerobic performance variations in elite soccer players. J Strength Cond Res 25(6):1502–1507. https://doi.org/10.1519/JSC.0b013e3181da85a9

Kannas TM, Amiridis IG, Arabatzi F, Katis A, Kellis E (2015) Changes in specific jumping performance after detraining period. J Sports Med Phys Fitness 55(10):1150–1156

Kellmann M, Bertollo M, Bosquet L, Brink M, Coutts AJ, Duffield R, Erlacher D, Halson SL, Hecksteden A, Heidari J, Kallus KW, Meeusen R, Mujika I, Robazza C, Skorski S, Venter R, Beckmann J (2018) Recovery and performance in sport: consensus statement. Int J Sports Physiol Perform 13(2):240–245. https://doi.org/10.1123/ijspp.2017-0759

Kenttä G, Hassmén P (1998) Overtraining and recovery. Sports Med 26(1):1–16. https://doi.org/10.2165/00007256-199826010-00001

Krustrup P, Mohr M, Amstrup T, Rysgaard T, Johansen J, Steensberg A, Pedersen PK, Bangsbo J (2003) The Yo-Yo intermittent recovery test: physiological response, reliability, and validity. Med Sci Sports Exerc 35(4):697–705. https://doi.org/10.1249/01.MSS.0000058441.94520.32

Lacome M, Simpson B, Buchheit M (2018) Monitoring training status with player-tracking technology. In: Still on the road to Rome part 1, vol 7, pp 55–63

Lambert MI, Borresen J (2010) Measuring training load in sports. Int J Sports Physiol Perform 5(3):406–411. https://doi.org/10.1123/ijspp.5.3.406

López-Segovia M, Dellal A, Chamari K, González-Badillo JJ (2014) Importance of muscle power variables in repeated and single sprint performance in soccer players. J Hum Kinet 40(1):201–211. https://doi.org/10.2478/hukin-2014-0022

Matveyev L (1981) Fundamentals of sports training. Progress Publishers

McCall A, Carling C, Nedelec M, Davison M, le Gall F, Berthoin S, Dupont G (2014) Risk factors, testing and preventative strategies for non-contact injuries in professional football: current perceptions and practices of 44 teams from various premier leagues. Br J Sports Med 48(18):1352–1357. https://doi.org/10.1136/bjsports-2014-093439

McGuigan M (2017) Monitoring training and performance in athletes. In: Monitoring training and performance in athletes. Human Kinetics

McLaren SJ, Macpherson TW, Coutts AJ, Hurst C, Spears IR, Weston M (2018) The relationships between internal and external measures of training load and intensity in team sports: a meta-analysis. Sports Med 48(3):641–658. https://doi.org/10.1007/s40279-017-0830-z

McMorris T, Barwood M, Hale BJ, Dicks M, Corbett J (2018) Cognitive fatigue effects on physical performance: a systematic review and meta-analysis. Physiol Behav 188:103–107. https://doi.org/10.1016/j.physbeh.2018.01.029

Miguel M, Oliveira R, Loureiro N, García-Rubio J, Ibáñez SJ (2021) Load measures in training/match monitoring in soccer: a systematic review. Int J Environ Res Public Health 18(5):2721. https://doi.org/10.3390/ijerph18052721

Morin J-B, le Mat Y, Osgnach C, Barnabò A, Pilati A, Samozino P, di Prampero PE (2021) Individual acceleration-speed profile in-situ: a proof of concept in professional football players. J Biomech 123:110524. https://doi.org/10.1016/j.jbiomech.2021.110524

Nagahara R, Morin J-B, Koido M (2016) Impairment of sprint mechanical properties in an actual soccer match: a pilot study. Int J Sports Physiol Perform 11(7):893–898. https://doi.org/10.1123/ijspp.2015-0567

Newton MD, Owen AL, Baker JS (2019) Monitoring external and internal training loads: relationships with injury risk in professional soccer: a review. EC Orthopaedic 10(9):686–697

Oliva-Lozano JM, Barbier X, Fortes V, Muyor JM (2021a) Key load indicators and load variability in professional soccer players: a full season study. Res Sports Med 1–13:201. https://doi.org/10.1080/15438627.2021.1954517

Oliva-Lozano JM, Gómez-Carmona CD, Rojas-Valverde D, Fortes V, Pino-Ortega J (2021b) Effect of training day, match, and length of the microcycle on the worst-case scenarios in professional soccer players. Res Sports Med 1–14:425. https://doi.org/10.1080/15438627.2021.1895786

Parmar N, James N, Hearne G, Jones B (2018) Using principal component analysis to develop performance indicators in professional rugby league. Int J Perform Anal Sport 18(6):938–949. https://doi.org/10.1080/24748668.2018.1528525

Pyne D, Martin D (2011) Fatigue—insights from individual and team sports. In: Regulation of fatigue in exercise, pp 177–186

Rabbani A, Kargarfard M, Twist C (2020) Fitness monitoring in elite soccer players: group vs. individual analyses. J Strength Cond Res 34(11):3250–3257. https://doi.org/10.1519/JSC.0000000000002700

Rago V (2019) Training load monitoring in football—application of field systems in professional male players, vol 55, p 703

Robertson S, Bartlett JD, Gastin PB (2017) Red, amber, or green? Athlete monitoring in team sport: the need for decision-support systems. Int J Sports Physiol Perform 12(s2):S2-73-S2-79. https://doi.org/10.1123/ijspp.2016-0541

Rossi A, Pappalardo L, Cintia P, Iaia FM, Fernàndez J, Medina D (2018) Effective injury forecasting in soccer with GPS training data and machine learning. PLoS One 13(7):e0201264. https://doi.org/10.1371/journal.pone.0201264

Rowell AE, Aughey RJ, Hopkins WG, Stewart AM, Cormack SJ (2017) Identification of sensitive measures of recovery after external load from football match play. Int J Sports Physiol Perform 12(7):969–976. https://doi.org/10.1123/ijspp.2016-0522

Ryan S, Kempton T, Coutts AJ (2021) Data reduction approaches to athlete monitoring in professional Australian football. Int J Sports Physiol Perform 16(1):59–65. https://doi.org/10.1123/ijspp.2020-0083

Saw AE, Main LC, Gastin PB (2016) Monitoring the athlete training response: subjective self-reported measures trump commonly used objective measures: a systematic review. Br J Sports Med 50(5):281–291. https://doi.org/10.1136/bjsports-2015-094758

Schneider C, Hanakam F, Wiewelhove T, Döweling A, Kellmann M, Meyer T, Pfeiffer M, Ferrauti A (2018) Heart rate monitoring in team sports—a conceptual framework for contextualizing heart rate measures for training and recovery prescription. Front Physiol 9:639. https://doi.org/10.3389/fphys.2018.00639

Schwellnus M, Soligard T, Alonso J-M, Bahr R, Clarsen B, Dijkstra HP, Gabbett TJ, Gleeson M, Hägglund M, Hutchinson MR, Janse Van Rensburg C, Meeusen R, Orchard JW, Pluim BM, Raftery M, Budgett R, Engebretsen L (2016) How much is too much? (part 2) International Olympic Committee consensus statement on load in sport and risk of illness. Br J Sports Med 50(17):1043–1052. https://doi.org/10.1136/bjsports-2016-096572

Scott BR, Lockie RG, Knight TJ, Clark AC, Janse de Jonge XAK (2013) A comparison of methods to quantify the in-season training load of professional soccer players. Int J Sports Physiol Perform 8(2):195–202. https://doi.org/10.1123/ijspp.8.2.195

Soligard T, Schwellnus M, Alonso J-M, Bahr R, Clarsen B, Dijkstra HP, Gabbett T, Gleeson M, Hägglund M, Hutchinson MR, Janse van Rensburg C, Khan KM, Meeusen R, Orchard JW, Pluim BM, Raftery M, Budgett R, Engebretsen L (2016) How much is too much? (part 1) International Olympic Committee consensus statement on load in sport and risk of injury. Br J Sports Med 50(17):1030–1041. https://doi.org/10.1136/bjsports-2016-096581

Starling LT, Lambert MI (2018) Monitoring Rugby players for fitness and fatigue: what do coaches want? Int J Sports Physiol Perform 13(6):777–782. https://doi.org/10.1123/ijspp.2017-0416

Taylor KL, Chapman DW, Cronin JB, Newton MJ, Gill ND (2012) Fatigue monitoring in high performance sport: a survey of current trends. J Aust Strength Cond 20:12–23

Thornton HR, Delaney JA, Duthie GM, Dascombe BJ (2019) Developing athlete monitoring systems in team sports: data analysis and visualization. Int J Sports Physiol Perform 14(6):698–705. https://doi.org/10.1123/ijspp.2018-0169

Thorpe RT, Strudwick AJ, Buchheit M, Atkinson G, Drust B, Gregson W (2015) Monitoring fatigue during the in-season competitive phase in elite soccer players. Int J Sports Physiol Perform 10(8):958–964. https://doi.org/10.1123/ijspp.2015-0004

Vanrenterghem J, Nedergaard NJ, Robinson MA, Drust B (2017) Training load monitoring in team sports: a novel framework separating physiological and biomechanical load-adaptation pathways. Sports Med 47(11):2135–2142. https://doi.org/10.1007/s40279-017-0714-2

Viru A, Viru M (2000) Nature of training effects. In: Garret W, Kirkendall D (eds) Exercise and sport science. Lippincott Williams & Williams, pp 67–95

Weaving D, Dalton NE, Black C, Darrall-Jones J, Phibbs PJ, Gray M, Jones B, Roe GAB (2018) The same story or a unique novel? Within-participant principal-component analysis of measures of training load in professional Rugby union skills training. Int J Sports Physiol Perform 13(9):1175–1181. https://doi.org/10.1123/ijspp.2017-0565

Wehbe GM, Hartwig TB, Duncan CS (2014) Movement analysis of Australian National league soccer players using global positioning system technology. J Strength Cond Res 28(3):834–842. https://doi.org/10.1519/JSC.0b013e3182a35dd1

Williams S, Trewartha G, Cross MJ, Kemp SPT, Stokes KA (2017) Monitoring what matters: a systematic process for selecting training-load measures. Int J Sports Physiol Perform 12(s2):S2-101-S2-106. https://doi.org/10.1123/ijspp.2016-0337

<u>GPSR Compliance</u>

The European Union's (EU) General Product Safety Regulation (GPSR) is a set of rules that requires consumer products to be safe and our obligations to ensure this.

If you have any concerns about our products, you can contact us on ProductSafety@springernature.com

In case Publisher is established outside the EU, the EU authorized representative is:

Springer Nature Customer Service Center GmbH
Europaplatz 3
69115 Heidelberg, Germany

Batch number: 10732119

Printed by Printforce, the Netherlands